Medical Mimics of Psychiatric Disorders

The
PROGRESS IN PSYCHIATRY
Series

David Spiegel, M.D.,
Series Editor

Medical Mimics of Psychiatric Disorders

Edited by
Irl Extein, M.D. and
Mark S. Gold, M.D.

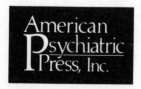

American Psychiatric Press, Inc.

1400 K Street, N.W.
Washington, DC 20005

Note: The authors have worked to ensure that all information in this book concerning drug dosages, schedules, and routes of administration is accurate as of the time of publication and consistent with standards set by the U.S. Food and Drug Administration and the general medical community. As medical research and practice advance, however, therapeutic standards may change. For this reason and because human and mechanical errors sometimes occur, we recommend that readers follow the advice of a physician who is directly involved in their care or the care of a member of their family.

Copyright © 1986 American Psychiatric Press, Inc.
ALL RIGHTS RESERVED
Manufactured in the United States of America

The paper used in this publication meets the minimum requirements of American National Standard for Information Sciences—Permanence of Paper for Printed Library Materials, ANSI Z39.48-1984.   ∞™

Library of Congress Cataloging in Publication Data

Medical mimics of psychiatric disorders.

(The Progress in psychiatry series)
Includes bibliographies.
1. Mental illness—Physiological aspects.
2. Psychological manifestations of general diseases.
3. Diagnosis, Differential. I. Extein, Irl, 1948–
II. Gold, Mark S., 1949–
III. Series. [DNLM: 1. Diagnosis, Differential.
2. Mental Disorders—diagnosis. WM 141 M489]
RC455.4.B5M43   1986   616'.047   86-8012
ISBN 0-88048-092-0 (alk. paper)

Contents

Contributors

R. Michael Allen, M.D.
Psychiatric Institute of Fort Worth, Fort Worth, Texas

Jeffrey R. Berlant, M.D.
Langley Porter Neuropsychiatric Institute, University of California School of Medicine, San Francisco, California

Linda Bierer, M.D.
Biological Psychiatry Branch, National Institute of Mental Health, Bethesda, Maryland

Charles A. Dackis, M.D.
Associate Director, Neuropsychiatric Evaluation Unit, Fair Oaks Hospital, Summit, New Jersey

Todd Wilk Estroff, M.D.
Research Facilities, Fair Oaks Hospital, Summit, New Jersey

Irl Extein, M.D.
Medical Director, Fair Oaks Hospital at Boca/Delray, Delray Beach, Florida

Barry S. Fogel, M.D.
Director, Inpatient Psychiatry, Rhode Island Hospital and Women & Infants Hospital; Consultant Psychiatrist, Roger Williams General Hospital; and Assistant Professor of Psychiatry, Brown University

Frederick C. Goggans, M.D.
Psychiatric Institute of Fort Worth, Fort Worth, Texas

Mark S. Gold, M.D.
Director of Research, Fair Oaks Hospital at Boca/Delray, Delray Beach, Florida

David A. Gross, M.D.
Clinical Director, Fair Oaks Hospital at Boca/Delray, Delray Beach, Florida

Russell T. Joffe, M.D.
Biological Psychiatry Branch, National Institute of Mental Health, Bethesda, Maryland

Robert M. Post, M.D.
Biological Psychiatry Branch, National Institute of Mental Health, Bethesda, Maryland

A. L. C. Pottash, M.D.
Executive Medical Director, Fair Oaks Hospital at Boca/Delray, Delray
Beach, Florida

Victor I. Reus, M.D.
Langley Porter Neuropsychiatric Institute, University of California School
of Medicine, San Francisco, California

Andrew E. Slaby, M.D., Ph.D., M.P.H.
Psychiatrist-in-Chief, Rhode Island Hospital and Women & Infants
Hospital; Director of Psychiatry, Roger Williams General Hospital;
and Professor of Psychiatry and Human Behavior, Brown University

Thomas W. Uhde, M.D.
Biological Psychiatry Branch, National Institute of Mental Health,
Bethesda, Maryland

Introduction to the *Progress in Psychiatry Series*

The *Progress in Psychiatry* Series is designed to capture in print the excitement that comes from assembling a diverse group of experts from various locations to examine in detail the newest information about a developing aspect of psychiatry. This series emerged as a collaboration between the American Psychiatric Association's Scientific Program Committee and the American Psychiatric Press, Inc. Great interest was generated by a number of the symposia presented each year at the APA Annual Meeting, and we realized that much of the information presented there, carefully assembled by people who are deeply immersed in a given area, would unfortunately not appear together in print. The symposia sessions at the Annual Meetings provide an unusual opportunity for experts who otherwise might not meet on the same platform to share their diverse viewpoints for a period of three hours. Some new themes are repeatedly reinforced and gain credence, while in other instances disagreements emerge, enabling the audience and now the reader to reach informed decisions about new directions in the field. The *Progress in Psychiatry* Series allows us to publish and capture some of the best of the symposia and thus provide an in-depth treatment of specific areas which might not otherwise be presented in broader review formats.

The symposia are selected on the basis of review by the Symposium Subcommittee of the Scientific Program Committee. From the approximately 80 symposia a year selected for presentation at the Annual Meeting, we choose approximately 10 percent which are deemed to be of especially high quality and to have interest to readers as well as meeting participants. After review by the American Psychiatric Press, we invite the authors to submit their papers as manuscripts for publication. We make every effort to expedite the publishing process so that books in the *Progress in Psychiatry* Series will be available as close as possible to the time of presentation at the Annual Meeting.

We believe the *Progress in Psychiatry* Series will provide you with an opportunity to review timely new information in specific fields of interest as they are developing. We hope you find that the excitement of the presentations is captured in the written word and that this book proves to be informative and enjoyable reading.

David Spiegel, M.D.
Series Editor
Progress in Psychiatry Series

Chapter 1

The Psychiatrist as Physician

David A. Gross, M.D.
Irl Extein, M.D.
Mark S. Gold, M.D.

Chapter 1

The Psychiatrist as Physician

Psychiatry's interest in the medical mimickers that produce counterfeit psychiatric syndromes reflects a long-standing guilt. This guilt stems from a renewed recognition of our collective ignorance of the functions of the human brain. In fact, Freud (1) may have set the stage for this guilt when he asserted that brain chemical dysfunction would provide an explanation for much behavioral pathology. Freud's followers may have unwittingly utilized denial and rationalization while spinning their complex web of psychodynamic theorems. These theorems were used to explain patients' maladaptive styles that were believed to be generated in response to the vicissitudes of everyday life. Like the proverb "you can't judge a book by its cover," psychiatric symptomatology may not signify psychiatric (psychodynamic) pathology.

Medical history has been replete with case studies that have called our attention to the relationship between physiology and behavior. Neurosyphilis fooled us for years, masquerading as *general paresis of the insane* (2) because of the presence of psychotic, depressive, manic, and schizophreniform symptomatology. This disease was called "insanity" for years. The "madness" component of *myxedema madness* (3) distracted clinicians from detecting the underlying thyroid endocrinopathy. It was the madness that struck us as the critical factor and blinded us from looking beyond the patient's mental state to the presence of pathophysiology. Regressing even further, the burning of "witches" to rid Salem of its "possessed" inhabitants was at that time a more apparent solution than considering that the individuals concerned might be displaying an epileptiform state (4).

Why is it, then, that the understanding of psychiatric illnesses and those individuals afflicted with such illnesses has led to clinical evaluative and treatment models that, until recently, have remained outside of the medical model? It has been known for a long time that the mind-body paradigm (5) represents a dichotomy that must be included in the psychiatric evaluation. This dichotomy has been clarified so that we now recognize that the brain does indeed mediate

3

behavior. Brain-behavior relationships are now better understood and more easily described. Body-brain and brain-body influences have been demonstrated and more clearly defined. So what has prevented a more rapid acceptance and application of the biological underpinnings of psychiatric disease?

Part of the answer to this question lies in the nature of the central nervous system (CNS) itself. The brain is a relatively inaccessible organ for study. The compactness, complexity, and indispensibility of cerebral components prevent easy scrutiny. To make matters worse, the major product of this organ, behavior, is extraordinarily difficult to describe and to measure. Fortunately, psychometric testing, behavior rating scales, electron microscopy, invasive and noninvasive radiologic imaging techniques, and neurochemical assaying have made the mystery of brain structure and function less and less obscure.

However, there is a uniqueness to the study of disorders of the mind compared to the study of disorders of other systems. The rate of advancement of our understanding of endocrinology, gastroenterology, cardiology, and so on has far exceeded similar progress in behavioral science. Clearly, ignorance alone has not been responsible for this knowledge disparity.

ATTITUDES AND BELIEF SYSTEMS

Perhaps one of the greatest obstacles to a more biologically oriented approach to psychiatric illness has been the attitudes and belief systems of Western society, which equates biologic causality with determinism. To some, determinism implies the presence of constitutional "weakness." The latter belief suggests that the problem is the result of the will of God (6) or a consequence of nature. Our society clearly prefers the tabula rasa pronouncements of John Locke (7). Belief in free will is a more palatable and optimistic approach to life than the pessimistic permanence that cellular damage implies.

Thus it may not be in the service of our attitudinal systems to consider the presence of biological dysfunction in our patients despite the fact that such dysfunction may be responsive to somatic treatment. When we prescribe a pill for a specified illness we are telling our patients that they have a biological abnormality. Furthermore, pill-taking implies that they cannot exercise their free will to rid themselves of this problem. All of us would prefer to view our bodies as indestructible products of creation or nature, allowing us unlimited potential and the freedom to maximize this potential willfully. The prescription of a medication directly or indirectly limits our degrees of freedom and narrows our reservoir of free will. It is no surprise that medication noncompliance poses problems for all medical disciplines. No one wants to accept the notion that they are "damaged goods" and it is exactly that type of attitude adjustment that successful pharmacotherapy compliance requires. Our patients must accept, as must we, the reality that 1) we are not born with perfect bodily machinery, 2) the machinery we inherit has limitations beyond which it breaks down, and 3) pathophysiological dysfunction of body parts develops over time as the result of natural biological clocks or acquired disease or insult.

We are suggesting that attitudinal adjustment of our society has been one of the necessary prerequisites for the advancement of general biological psychiatry. We are only beginning to be able to accept the belief that cellular pathology may underlie abnormalities of mentation and mood. The novel idea that organic processes may require initial stabilization before ideational therapy becomes efficacious is relatively new to psychiatry. Many mental health clinicians still believe that the primary function of pharmacotherapy is to facilitate psychotherapy. Psychotherapy cannot be ignored as a treatment modality, but it cannot remain as the primary treatment option of choice.

Treatment choice clearly depends on diagnosis. Psychiatric diagnoses have traditionally been derived from a psychosocial data base. From a free will perspective, one can see how it would be more acceptable to consider psychological or social causality. Psychosocial therapeutic manipulation becomes consonant with free will expression because the patient is guided along the path toward recovery by the therapist. The therapist fosters and shapes the patient's "natural" expression of free will. At the same time, lack of therapeutic progress can be understood as resistance to this process and an inability to maximize free will potential.

A psychosociobiological model utilizing a general systems approach (8) allows for the incorporation of the dependent variables that may influence the illness state. Furthermore, appropriate weights can be applied to the more critical variables. For example, the depressed individual with occult hypothyroidism and marital discord cannot be adequately assessed until one has accounted for the endocrinopathy. Continuation of depressive signs and symptoms in this case despite adequate thyroid replacement suggests that a greater diagnostic weight must be attached to the psychosocial variable. The addition of an abnormal dexamethasone suppression test and signs of major affective illness (9) further adds a neurochemical CNS factor.

It is therefore not unreasonable to investigate systematically the psychosociobiological systems as part of any modern neuropsychiatric evaluation. This approach requires that the psychiatrist accept the poorly differentiated phenomenology of psychiatric syndromes and aggressively search for biological causality. A preconceived belief that mental state findings are the direct result of psychodynamic conflicts obfuscates the ability to detect the brain-body mechanisms that all too often are critically responsible for symptom development. Psychic complaints actively reflect brain operation. Brain function or dysfunction reflects the intra- and extraneurocellular homeostatic milieu that in and of itself is influenced by the extra-CNS (body) biochemical environment. The myriad subtle biological variables influencing behavior will be overlooked unless we seek them out. This investigatory process requires a conscious intent on our part and the tools of modern technology. Renovation of the *Diagnostic and Statistical Manual of Mental Disorders*, Third Edition (DSM-III) (9) has been one product of attitudinal change.

DSM-III

A major problem with the DSM-III is that it invokes a rational, decision-tree oriented and factor analytic format that can lull the unwary clinician into a false sense of diagnostic security. We may come to believe that we have utilized a tight scientific approach in ruling-in a DSM-III diagnosis. However, as the DSM-III points out, we are utilizing a descriptive, not an etiologic, nosology. Perhaps future DSM editions will provide specific decision-tree methodology for ruling-out the medical causes of psychiatric phenomenology. We need more sophistication and training in ruling-out medical illness before we can be expected to decide on primary psychiatric etiology.

How can psychiatry accomplish the tasks of ruling-out medical illness? Traditionally this task has been assigned to the medical–surgical consultants called in to see our patients. This arrangement has a number of inherent problems. First, the presence of a psychiatric patient colors the consultant's evaluation. Consultants share in the problem of attitude and belief system adjustment described previously. Because of the presence of abnormal and often bizarre mental states, psychiatric patients may instill a generalized uneasiness in consultants. An opinion poll of consultants called to see a psychiatric patient with abdominal pain as compared to cancer patients with abdominal pain would probably reveal greater comfort and empathy with the latter patient population than with the former.

The attitudes described are basic to the human psyche: we avoid what is different and hard to understand. We are comfortable with what we can explain, predict, and control. That is not to say that this editorial comment on the consultation process is universal. The medical–surgical consultant who demonstrates an acute understanding of the complexities involved in consulting to the psychiatric patient will spend more time and effort because such a consult is generally more difficult. The data base is more difficult to objectify because the ability of psychiatric patients to give a medical history may be impaired by the presence of their mental state aberrations. Laboratory testing and careful complete physical examination are often more important and fundamental to the consultation process.

We have erroneously kept referring to the individuals being treated as *our patients* or *psychiatric patients*. In reality they are *our mutual patients* when it turns out that the true cause for their psychic-behavioral distress is medical. This faux pas is part of the problem; it is too easy to label patients with psychiatric patienthood. Our attitudes support these labels and so do our insecurities. The patient with chronic abdominal pain, DSM-III criteria for major depression, and a non-specific physical examination and laboratory screening becomes a psychiatric patient for want of a better diagnosis. This decision-tree outcome is reached because we may have yet to uncover our patient's pancreatic neoplasm and have difficulty accepting the possibility that the diagnosis has evaded us. Moreover, because every physician is indoctrinated to relieve suffering, the patient described will be a medical treatment failure if the consulting physician truly believes that the yet-to-be-discovered etiology is medical. Suffering cannot be relieved unless treatment can be directed at something. Thus this untenable position is avoided by passing the locus of control back to the psychiatrist and recommending that the only treatment necessary is psychiatric.

This dilemma is not beyond solution. As important as it is to guide the psychiatrist back toward a medical model and differential diagnostic approach toward patients, it is incumbent on psychiatry to maximize the effectiveness of the medical evaluation. This requires that the medical consultant must be incorporated into the psychiatric treatment team. It is our job to work with the medical consultant during the consultation process so that the impediments toward finding a medical etiology are avoided and a medical diagnosis can be confidently ruled out.

The challenge to the American Psychiatric Association and future editions of the DSM is clear. Descriptive nosology must be complemented by an etiologic, evaluative process that allows for specific psychiatric diagnosis by biologic inclusion rather than exclusion. There must be more specificity in the DSM than merely the ruling-out of medical causality in order to be able to rule-in primary psychiatric disease.

TECHNOLOGY AND REALITY TESTING

Society's greater acceptance of mental disease may be a by-product of the rapid expansion of scientific methodology and equipment. Although one could support a "chicken or egg" dichotomy, neurobiology's technological advances have been responsible for many of the attitudinal adjustments so long awaited in modern psychiatric circles. We are amassing hard, incontrovertible evidence for the role of brain-body interactions in the production of psychiatric symptomatology. Previous speculative assumptions can no longer be ignored. Acceptance has become the rule. We now talk about brain neurotransmitters, neuroregulators, neuromodulators, pre- and post-synaptic up-and-down regulation, GABA-benzodiazepine chloride ionophore receptor complexes, and so on. We even recognize the role of extra-CNS secretagogues like cholecystokinin, testosterone, thyroxine, and endorphins on CNS function. Autonomous electrical discharges in critical regions of the temporal lobes are now believed to be responsible for a wide spectrum of psychiatric symptomatology (10). The kindling model (11) in cats and monkeys has provided a paradigm for the enduring neurophysiological effects of electrical and chemical (12) stimulation of the brain. These intriguing studies raise the possibility that adult CNS circuitry is more malleable than previously thought and that lasting behavioral change may in actuality reflect persistent structure-function alterations. An animal model for opiate withdrawal has led to the use of the alpha agonist clonidine in blocking the brain stem mediation of withdrawal in heroin addicts (13). The ability to provoke artificially the hypothalamic-pituitary-adrenal axis with dexamethasone or the hypothalamic-pituitary-thyroid axis with thyrotropin-releasing hormone (14) has resulted in clarification of affective illness diagnosis in the former and the unmasking of hypothyroidism in the latter.

The above would not be possible without the availability of the modern psychiatric laboratory. Liquid and gas chromatography, ultracentrifugation, radioimmunochemistry, and mass spectroscopy have permitted the psychiatric clinician access to brain-body relationships previously denied. Most importantly, computer analysis has mushroomed our data base and accelerated the transition from laboratory experiment to clinical application. Computer availability has permitted the clinical psychiatrist research design capabilities without requiring a large research team. Research-quality clinical neurochemistry laboratories with 24-hour turnaround courier service add a most important link to the chain between speculative neuroscience and the clinical practice of psychiatry. Diagnostic hypotheses can be ruled-in and ruled-out, blood levels and dose-response characteristics of psychotropic agents tracked, and biological markers like DST, 3-methyoxy-4-hydroxyphenylglycol can be studied to help predict treatment response and failure and relapse risks.

These practical technological advances have provided psychiatry with the reality testing necessary for successful entrance into the 1980s. The mind-brain-body trichotomy of past decades can no longer be rigidly utilized for the understanding of psychiatric illnesses. The technological revolution has fostered the attitudinal evolution that participated in the successful application of the biopsychosocial model. It is no longer heresy for a clinician to consider first the biological system in a patient with psychiatric symptoms. For example, a psychotic mental state in a young individual no longer reflexly leads to the diagnosis of schizophrenia. Evaluation of this patient requires a comprehensive search for the varied and often reversible medical mimics of the psychotic state and includes drug, toxin, and heavy metal screens; electroencephalogram; computerized axial tomography; neuropsychological testing; and comprehensive blood chemistry batteries. Similarly, multiple sclerosis, often presenting in its early stages with paramount psychiatric stigmata, had been most difficult to diagnose until nuclear magnetic resonance scanning made it easier to detect demyelinating plaques. Of course, a sophisticated technological armamentarium must be guided by a therapeutic doctor–patient relationship.

DIAGNOSIS RELATED GROUPS AND ECONOMICS

The coupling of technological progress with attitudinal change has not come too soon for American psychiatry. Economic and political realities now dictate the practice of medicine. The care of patients with mental illnesses is no exception. General hospital budgets are being scrutinized while state mental health department programs are being curtailed. State hospital capacity has been drastically reduced with the deinstitutionalization program. All of this has transpired in the absence of any unified or planned community mental health program. To make matters worse, state financial mental health and social services have been severely limited by the paucity of federal funding and the redistribution of local monies.

What does this mean for the practice of general psychiatry? Budgetary restraints and insufficient number of psychiatric beds have necessitated a shortening of the length of a patient's hospital stay. In many instances this has resulted in premature discharge of the patient and subsequent readmission. The revolving door syndrome for chronic psychiatric patients continues, not necessarily the product of inadequate diagnosis and treatment but quite often the result of limited time to establish definitive diagnostic and treatment plans.

The federal government has attempted to solve this problem for the nonpsychiatric medical–surgical patient by designing the prospective payment system of diagnosis related groups (DRGs). A patient's illness is reimbursed prospectively based on a national or regional schedule. Hospital costs accrued beyond the predicted cost (or length of stay) must be absorbed by the hospital. Medical and surgical disciplines have responded to this challenge by becoming more efficient in evaluative work-ups and acute treatment. More definitive and cost effective laboratory protocols are being utilized. More than ever, physicians are becoming aware of what tests get what for their money.

Prospective payment systems are ready and waiting for psychiatry. Is psychiatry prepared for prospective payment? To meet the demands of prospective payment and DRGs, psychiatric hospital units must:

1. Learn to develop rapidly an objective and meaningful data base for newly admitted patients. The neuropsychiatric evaluation unit model performs this function admirably.
2. Utilize the staff multidisciplinary evaluative team to produce a comprehensive master plan. This specially trained and supervised staff orchestrates the neuropsychiatric interviews, psychosocial evaluation, neuroendocrine and other laboratory testing, electroencephalography, neuropsychological testing, psychiatric rating scales, and medical consultations that contribute to the treatment plan.
3. Rapidly engage the staff multidisciplinary team in the treatment of the critical biopsychosocial systems variables that have been defined by evaluation of the data base as responsible for the psychiatric illness. Treatment that begins on the evaluation unit leads to more rapid discharge from the treatment unit. Relapse risk is reduced along with length of stay.
4. Carefully prescribe postdischarge treatment plans to maintain stability and prevent relapse.

Biological system dysfunction can often present the most critical treatment variables. For example, psychosociotherapy of the highest order for the depressed individual will be for naught unless the hypothyroidism is treated. Likewise, social skills and assertiveness training will not effectively help the patient with partial complex seizure-mediate panic anxiety and depersonalization symptoms. Similarly, the DRG lengths of stay for major depressive illness will be adversely influenced by tricyclic noncompliance or inadequate response. Use of clinical laboratory tricyclic assays in dose-prediction testing enables efficient early determination of drug metabolism (15) and consequently favorably influences length of hospitalization. Thus an intensive and complete biological evaluation must parallel the psychosocial data collection. Neuropsychiatric examination and laboratory testing become the mainstay of this approach.

CONCLUSION

The challenge of the 1980s is upon psychiatry. We can no longer rely on intrapsychic conflicts as the explanation for psychiatric illness. Moreover, technological advances make it difficult to ignore the interrelationships between mental state and brain function. Our knowledge of this interaction must expand to include other body systems. The more we understand the physiological bases of abnormal behavior, the more the medical mimics of psychiatric disorders become meaningful. This enlightenment has resulted in narrowing of the spectrum of true psychiatric disease.

It would seem that this situation might limit the role of the psychiatrist. But this is not the case if the psychiatrist accepts the role of the primary physician responsible for the review of all systems: biological, psychological, and social. The psychiatrist's use of the medical model in the evaluation and treatment of patients becomes essential. A solid grounding in neuroscience complemented by a healthy dose of clinical curiosity and investigative diligence contribute to the making of a modern psychiatrist. These assets must be backed by a modern, research-capable neurochemistry laboratory. Finally, the utilization of a multidisciplinary team for hospital-based neuropsychiatric evaluation and treatment adds a critical dimension to the cost effective and scientific demands of an expanding specialty.

REFERENCES

1. Brenner C: An Elementary Textbook of Psychoanalysis. New York, International Universities Press, 1974, p 16

2. Bruetsch WL: Neurosyphilitic conditions: general paralysis, general paresis, dementia paralytica, in American Handbook of Psychiatry, Vol. 4. Edited by Reiser MF. New York, Basic Books, 1975, pp 134–151

3. Whybrow PC, Prang AJ, Treadway CR: Mental changes accompanying thyroid gland dysfunction. Arch Gen Psychiatry 20:48–63, 1969

4. Mora G: Historical and theoretical trends in psychiatry, in Comprehensive Textbook of Psychiatry. Edited by Freedman AM, Kaplan HI, Sadock BJ. Baltimore, Williams & Wilkins Co, 1975

5. Dunbar HF: Mind and Body: Psychosomatic Medicine. New York, Random House, 1947

6. Smith CB: Makers of Modern Thought. New York, Heritage Publishing Co, 1972

7. Locke, J: An essay concerning human understanding, in The English Philosophers from Bacon to Mill. Edited by Burtt EA. New York, Random House, 1939

8. Gross DA: Medical origins of psychiatric emergencies. Int J Psychiatry Med 11(1):1–24, 1981–1982

9. American Psychiatric Association: Diagnostic and Statistical Manual of Mental Disorders. 3rd Ed. Washington, DC, American Psychiatric Association, 1980

10. Waxman SG, Geschwind N: The interictal behavior syndrome of temporal lobe epilepsy. Arch Gen Psychiatry 32:1590–1596, 1975

11. Goddard GV, McIntyre DC, Leech CK: A permanent change in brain function resulting from daily electrical stimulation. Exp Neurol 25:295–330, 1969

12. Post RM, Kopanda RT: Cocaine, kindling and psychosis. Am J Psychiatry 133:627–634, 1976

13. Gold MS, Redmond DE, Kleber HD: Noradrenergic hyperactivity in opiate withdrawal supported by clonidine reversal of opiate withdrawal. Am J Psychiatry 136:100, 1979

14. Extein I, Pottash ALC, Gold MS: TRH test in depression. N Engl J Med 302:923, 1980

15. Cooper TB, Simpson GM: Prediction of individual dosage of nortriptyline. Am J Psychiatry 135:333–335, 1978

Chapter 2

Neurological Screening of Psychiatric Patients

Barry S. Fogel, M.D.
Andrew E. Slaby, M.D., Ph.D., M.P.H.

Chapter 2

Neurological Screening of Psychiatric Patients

Psychiatric symptoms are nonspecific. They occur with medical and psychiatric illnesses and, in some instances, are harbingers of neurological disease. Hall et al. (1–3) and others (4, 5) have found in reviews of consecutive admissions to ambulatory and inpatient psychiatric services a high prevalence of concomitant medical illness. Often the physical illness is etiologically responsible for the psychiatric distress. At other times it contributes to the onset of psychiatric symptoms or results from the psychiatric illness or its treatment. Johnson (6) performed detailed physical examinations on 250 consecutive admissions to an inpatient psychiatric service and found 12 percent to be suffering from physical conditions that were a causative factor for the presenting psychiatric illness. Of these, 80 percent had been missed by a physician prior to admission and 6.6 percent were initially missed after admission. Of all patients admitted, 60 percent had abnormal physical findings.

Psychiatric symptoms may be caused by alcohol-related syndromes, degenerative brain diseases, cerebrovascular diseases, endocrinopathies, traumatic brain damage, collagen diseases, demyelinating brain diseases, seizures, encephalitides, and toxic and metabolic diseases (7–16). Recognizing physical illness should not be difficult when physical signs such as changes in reflexes, fever, or hemiparesis accompany the psychiatric symptoms. Problems arise when the symptoms are confined to alterations of mood, thought, or behavior, and when the neurologic signs are not evident unless specifically sought.

In this chapter we will suggest several ways for psychiatrists to screen their patients more effectively for neurologic disease, which may cause or contribute to psychiatric disorders. Our advice is based on extensive clinical experience in a general hospital setting, bolstered by critical review of the literature. We will elaborate on four main themes: 1) improving the neurologic examination, 2) understanding the specific diagnostic strengths of the electroencephalogram (EEG)

15

versus the computed tomography (CT) scan, 3) making the most of the EEG, and 4) improving the formulation of the neurologic differential diagnosis.

IMPROVING THE NEUROLOGIC EXAMINATION

The effectiveness of the psychiatrist's neurological examination increases when the neurological examination is viewed as a hypothesis-testing examination rather than as the routine application of a list of neurologic tests. The following three subsections elaborate on this point.

The sensitivity and specificity of neurological signs in the detection of occult organic brain disease depend on the clinical population and diseases suspected.   For instance, when multiple sclerosis is suspected, as it ought to be in "hysterics," bedside examination of eye movements may be insensitive to diagnostically relevant abnormalities. Measurement of eye movements in 84 patients with multiple sclerosis and 21 patients with optic neuritis using a simple portable electrophysiological apparatus revealed a subclinical eye movement disorder in 80 percent of the definite, 74 percent of the probable, and 60 percent of the possible multiple sclerosis patients (17). When subdural hematoma is suspected, as it ought to be when subacute mental status change occurs together with alcoholism, advanced age, or chronic headache, the little known and seldom practiced technique of auscultatory percussion may be remarkably sensitive and specific. Of 89 consecutive patients with suspected intracranial masses examined by auscultatory percussion and subsequent CT scan, 51 percent had positive findings on auscultation. Of these, 86 percent had positive findings on auscultation. Only 7 percent of the 27 patients with normal scans were false positive on percussion (18).

Auscultatory percussion is simple; we quote in full its description from the article that establishes its concurrent validity with the CT scan (18).

> The procedure is simple and requires only a stethoscope. The patient may be supine or, preferably, sitting with the head facing forward. The examiner faces the patient or stands on one side. Direct percussion is applied lightly and with equal intensity with the pulp of a finger at a marked point in the midline of the upper forehead well above the frontal sinuses, which extend about 3 cm above the superorbital ridge and have a breadth of about 2.5 cm. (Dullness is normal over the sinuses and could interfere with the examination.) The bell piece of the stethoscope is applied with the other hand on the head methodically and alternately from one side to the opposite side of the head at corresponding anatomical areas. (Changing hands is more comfortable for the examiner.) Differ-

ences in sound between the opposite sides of the head are compared. An imaginary horizontal plane across the upper borders of the helices of the ears extending bilaterally from the forehead to the occiput is a useful anatomical guide. The bell piece, preferably with a rubber rim, is applied on this plane beginning distal to the palpable vertical ridge on the side of the forehead and proceeding to the occiput. To avoid missing diseased areas successive applications of the stethoscope should not exceed the diameter of the bell piece. With the same technique, progressively higher planes toward the vertex are examined. The bell piece must be applied with complete contact and be evenly seated on the head; it may be applied directly to the hair without interference. Normally there is no difference in sound between both sides of the head. An intracranial mass lying in the path of the generated sound vibrations and their reception produces distinct dullness compared with the opposite side. Most of the abnormal findings have been detected in the frontoparietal temporal areas within a 6 cm plane above the helices of the ears. The difference in intensity of sound is often pronounced and in many patients may be detected quickly. It can be shown and measured by phonoscopy. With minimal practice and experience the examiner can become proficient and complete the examination within five minutes.

Tests infrequently performed may detect confirmatory evidence of an organically based disorder, whereas commonly used screening tests are often insensitive to psychiatrically relevant diffuse cerebral pathology. Jenkyn et al. (19) correlated evidence of diffuse cerebral disorder as measured by the Halstead Reitan Neuropsychological Battery with findings on neurological examination and found 13 physical signs with a false negative rate of less than 60 percent. These included the glabellar blink, the nuchocephalic reflex, the suck reflex, impairment of upward gaze, impairment of downward gaze, a tendency to keep the raised arm up after the signal to drop it, impaired visual tracking, impersistence of lateral gaze, trouble accurately recalling three items after a time delay with intervening distraction, paratonia of both arms, difficulty spelling "world" backwards, paratonia of both legs, and difficulty in giving past presidents in reverse order. By contrast, they found an extremely high false negative rate, over 85 percent for popularly used tests such as the Babinski sign, double simultaneous stimulation, orientation to place and date, and recall of current presidents.

The glabellar blink is elicited by rapidly tapping the patient's glabella with the examiner's index finger eight to ten times. A normal response is for reflex closure of the eyelids to cease after two or three taps; continued blinking is abnormal. The nuchocephalic reflex is elicited by briskly turning the shoulders of the patient to the left or right. A normal response is for the head to follow after a lag of about half a second. If the head does not turn to follow the shoulders, the response is abnormal. The test cannot be interpreted if neck disease leads to turning of the head and shoulders en bloc. Paratonia is an irregular resistance by the patient to the examiner's efforts to flex and extend the patient's limbs, despite instructions for the patient to relax. Spasticity and parkinsonian rigidity can be differentiated from paratonia by their typical pattern and by their greater consistency. For further details on these and other bedside tests of cerebral dysfunction, see Jenkyn et al. (19).

Enlarged pupils may be the only neurological sign in addition to the abnormal mental state in cases of anticholinergic delirium (20, 21). In these cases, vital signs are abnormal but somatic motor and reflex signs are absent. In many other acute confusional states that include cognitive, sensory, memory, and attentional aberrations, there are no focal or lateralizing sensory or motor signs because the neurological disorder is diffuse or multifocal.

Patients presenting with head trauma in the emergency setting are often unable to provide a history. In the presence of behavior compatible with a head injury, a psychiatrist must look for scalp wounds and indirect evidence of basal skull fractures, such as Battle's sign and cerebrospinal fluid otorrhea and rhinorrhea. (Battle's sign is bogginess of the temporal or postauricular region due to subcutaneous fluid or blood.) If not personally doing the physical examination, the psychiatrist must verify that the examiner has looked for these signs. X-rays of the neck, chest, and skull may be obtained. Amnesia for an accident with head injury is sufficient for diagnosis of concussion even if there is no history of loss of consciousness (22).

This last point deserves emphasis. Our experience in consulting to a busy regional trauma center suggests that evidence of concussion is not always sought by the trauma team when the patient arrives at the emergency room awake and other physical injuries need immediate care. The psychiatrist, if called afterwards for assessment of posttraumatic behavior changes, must make the diagnosis retrospectively from evidence of posttraumatic amnesia. If the patient is examined soon enough after the injury, anterograde amnesia may still be present. If it is, the presence of neurologic dysfunction is unequivocal.

The ability to communicate with gestures in the presence of muteness has no value in distinguishing functional from organic etiologies. A study of the 9 mute patients who occurred in 350 consecutive general hospital admissions for head injury revealed that all of the patients with mutism could communicate somewhat with gestures.

However, all who were tested showed impaired writing (23). All recovered some speech, although the 4 of the 9 patients with basal ganglia lesions made a less complete recovery. Unlike the ability to gesture, the ability to write a coherent sentence to dictation is, in general, a good high sensitivity screening test for organically based language disorder.

Specific visual examinations are superior to screening eye examinations. In a review of 18 patients with probable or definite multiple sclerosis and 20/20 vision (17), 16 had one or more abnormalities on other measures of ocular function, such as visual-evoked potentials and psychophysical tests of contrast sensitivity. Of these 16, 59 percent had pallor of the optic nerve head or changes in the nerve fiber layer on fundoscopy. Normal visual acuity does not exclude visual system disorder. Careful funduscopic examination is mandatory to screen the visual system properly. It should certainly be done in all patients suspected of multiple sclerosis, a group including all patients suspected of a conversion disorder with neurologic symptoms.

While we do not expect psychiatrists to be expert in all aspects of funduscopic examination, the determination of pallor of the optic nerve head is easy, and frequently has been valuable in differential diagnosis. Thus a reasonable set of skills for the psychiatrist would include examination of the optic disk, assessment of visual fields by confrontation, and assessment of visual accuity. Theoretical knowledge of other parts of the visual examination is helpful in assessing the completeness or incompleteness of screening done by other physicians. Even eye examinations by ophthalmologists may not include all of the relevant points for assessment of multiple sclerosis, unless the ophthalmologist is specifically asked by the psychiatrist to look for such evidence (24).

Gait disorder may be the only hard sign of a treatable neurological illness. Dubin et al. (16) studied 1,140 patients cleared medically on an emergency psychiatric service. Of these, 39 showed signs of disorientation, abnormal vital signs, or clouding of consciousness and, of these, 38 were found to have an organic disorder (one was diagnosed as paranoid schizophrenia). On review of initial history and physical examination, 14 of the 38 had gait disturbance, weight loss, hypertension, abnormal vital signs, or a significant medical history.

In a neurological evaluation of 50 patients over the age of 70 with gait disturbance of previously undetermined etiology, 24 percent had an illness that could either be treated or palliated (25). Specific observation of gait is helpful in the diagnosis of Parkinson's disease and cerebellar atrophy. Robins (26) contended that 10 to 33 percent of patients presenting for evaluation of dementia have a potentially reversible cause. A summary of six studies involving 503 patients revealed the leading causes of reversible dementia to be normal pressure hydrocephalus, depression, subdural hematoma or intracranial mass, other psychiatric disorders, drugs, and thyroid disease. The neurological conditions on this list may not produce focal motor or sensory signs, but may show only disturbances of mental status and gait. Normal pressure hydrocephalus virtually always affects gait.

For these reasons, examination of gait is essential in any complete psychiatric evaluation. Observation of the patient walking into a room and taking a seat is an easy, unobtrusive part of any psychiatric interview. If subtle abnormalities are noticed, they can be brought out by asking the patient to perform special tasks. Mild weakness of one side can be brought out by having the patient walk on tiptoes and on heels. The foot may droop on the weak side. Patients who appear slightly off balance can be asked to walk on an imaginary line, touching heel to toe, as in the familiar test for intoxication. Patients suspected of parkinsonism should be observed making turns, and on speeding up and slowing down to command. Finally, it is worth noting that involuntary movements and posturing of the arms are sometimes most evident when the patient is walking.

UNDERSTANDING THE SPECIFIC DIAGNOSTIC STRENGTHS OF THE EEG AND THE CT SCAN

The EEG, one of the earliest ancillary physiologic tests in psychiatry, remains one of the most useful in the clinical assessment of the psychiatric patient. Although it has been eclipsed in the public imagination by brain imaging, it is actually more useful in distinguishing functional from organic psychiatric symptoms in many circumstances. In addition, it is an inexpensive test readily available in many small hospitals without CT scanners, and in psychiatric hospitals with limited medical laboratory facilities.

The EEG detects abnormal brain function; the CT scan detects abnormal anatomy. While a CT scan would be essential to screen for brain metastases in a cancer patient with subacute mental changes, it would be less helpful in circumstances where no anatomical abnormality of the brain would be likely. For instance, in cases of reversible diffuse brain dysfunction on a toxic metabolic basis, the CT is normal while the EEG may be diagnostic. The detection of mild deliria presenting psychiatrically and the differentiation of pseudodementia from degenerative cerebral disease have been cited as two established indications for the use of the EEG in psychiatry (27).

Mild diffuse brain damage due to hypoxia and hypotension may contribute to psychiatric disorders following open heart surgery. The EEG may be the only laboratory evidence of such diffuse damage. In a study of 100 patients evaluated following open heart surgery for cardiac valvular disease, 38 thought to be neurologically asymptomatic received EEGs postoperatively; 14 showed abnormalities. In the same study, 15 of the 49 who received careful post-operative neuropsychological evaluation showed cognitive deficits. Yet only 4 of the 100 were diagnosed as cognitively disordered by their primary physicians (28). The "hard" abnormality of an abnormal EEG can be useful diagnostically in linking cognitive disorder to probable hypotensive injury.

Abnormal EEGs are found in two-thirds of untreated patients with pernicious anemia, and in virtually all with significant organic mental findings (29). Thus, in a patient with a psychiatric disorder and a low B12 level, the EEG might provide confirmatory evidence that the low B12 level was psychiatrically relevant. The CT scan would be of no value in such a situation. Herpes simplex encephalitis, which may present with nonspecific symptoms of psychiatric illness, may produce an abnormal EEG in an early stage while the CT is negative and the cerebrospinal fluid (CSF) is not diagnostic. Thus, in suspected cases, all three tests should be done, and the EEG should not be omitted even if the CT and CSF exams are normal (30).

The CT scan, while of dramatic relevance in identifying anatomic lesions of the brain, has not proved particularly valuable in clinical assessment of patients with psychiatric disorders not accompanied by other neurologic signs and symptoms, and not occurring in a setting highly suggestive of organic causation. CT scans performed on 46 patients (mean age 32) with acute psychoses and 46 healthy volunteers (mean age 27) showed that the patients as a group had wider third and lateral ventricles, but did not show any specific focal lesions in the psychotic group (31). In another study, CT scanning of 47 psychiatric patients referred with a clinical diagnosis of organic brain syndrome yielded two subdural hematomas and one infarct; the remainder had cerebral atrophy. Of 21 patients in the same study referred with gross neurological symptoms or signs accompanying their psychiatric disorder, the yield of specific abnormalities was higher and included an arachnoid cyst, an astrocytoma, a pituitary tumor, and two major hemisphere infarctions (32).

Thus the clinician should always consider a CT when the setting strongly suggests an anatomic focal lesion, as would be the case in a patient with known malignancy, known cerebrovascular disease, head trauma, and so on. For patients with dementia, a CT should be done to rule out subdural hematoma, normal pressure hydro-cephalus, meningioma, and other such treatable lesions. The patient with an acute or subacute mental status change and no focal signs in a nonsuspicious setting would probably be better screened with an EEG, with CT follow-up of focal EEG abnormalities, if any. Finally, in any case where the neuropsychiatric findings are atypical or puzzling, both an EEG and a CT probably will be necessary to diagnose the case properly.

The above remarks on the diagnostic limitations of the CT scan will probably need revision as techniques for interpreting subtle CT abnormalities become more reliable, and as evidence accumulates concerning the correlation between CT scan findings and outcome in the "functional" psychoses. There may come a time when CT or other brain imaging results may be useful for clinical management or assessment of prognosis in patients with schizophrenia or manic depressive illness. However, given the present state of the evidence, we would not currently recommend CT scans for this purpose.

MAKING THE MOST OF THE EEG

Brain electrical activity is a dynamic phenomenon that changes with time, circumstances, and the patient's state of arousal. The diagnostic efficacy of the EEG is greatest when the test is timed with this in mind. To take an obvious example, the patient who is said to awaken from sleep with brief episodes of bizarre behavior requires a sleep EEG to be properly investigated for nocturnal epilepsy, including, ideally, an all-night sleep study that could in addition assess the patient for abnormalities of sleep architecture. The following sub-sections elaborate on this theme.

EEGs are most valuable in the identification of organic brain disease when obtained when patients are symptomatic. A psychiatrist wish-ing to evaluate a neurological etiology for suspected paroxysmal hysterical or anxiety symptoms should not only obtain a routine EEG, but should also try to get one under the circumstances a patient feels will elicit an attack. Fariello et al. (33) reported on 32 cases of patients with paroxysmal symptoms who were studied as they reen-acted the situations that provoked their paroxysmal attacks while having simultaneous polygraphic recording of EEG, electrocardi-ogram, and respiration. They found it necessary to change the di-agnoses in 19 cases, many of which had been previously diagnosed as hysterical. Provocative circumstances included having patients take a bath, stand up quickly, read, and undergo venipuncture. A careful history and awareness of the existence of unusual seizure types is helpful in diagnosing epilepsy—for example, a "vibe" or "chill" (34)—

but ictal EEG abnormality during the time of the suspected seizure makes possible an unequivocal diagnosis.

An emergency EEG is a definitive procedure when partial complex status is expected. Nonconvulsive status epilepticus should be suspected in instances of acute mental status change with diminished responsiveness or automatic behavior, particularly in patients with a past history of seizures. Partial complex status may present as a confusional state, as aphasia, or as decreased responsiveness with staring. Although a history of seizures is often present, there are well-documented cases with no past history of epilepsy. The interictal EEG was abnormal in 8 cases reported by Ballenger et al. (35) and in 9 of the 12 cases reviewed from literature. The neurologic examination was normal in 4 of the 8 cases reported. But, the *ictal* EEG was abnormal in every case where it was performed.

Sleep EEGs, sleep-deprived EEGs, and EEGs with special leads may help with the diagnosis of temporal lobe epilepsy, but even with these procedures, the EEG may always be normal or nondiagnostic. Thus temporal lobe epilepsy remains a clinical diagnosis, to be established by a careful history, clinical observation, and, if necessary, therapeutic trials of anticonvulsants. Because the clinical manifestations of temporal lobe epilepsy may overlap with the manifestations of functional psychiatric disorders, psychiatric clinicians tend to attach great importance to the presence or absence of diagnostic EEG abnormalities.

Unfortunately, there are patients with definite temporal lobe epilepsy with no focal spike activity detectable, even with special leads. A typical case is included in a report on electrophysiological correlates of pathology and surgical results in temporal lobe epilepsy (36). A patient with no definite spike focus on scalp EEG or sphenoidal leads had a definite lateral temporal spike focus on electrocorticography. This patient had total relief of seizures following anterior temporal lobectomy; the pathology was medial temporal sclerosis.

Different authors disagree on the incidence of negative EEGs in temporal lobe epilepsy. Much of the disagreement may be explainable by differences in the clinical populations studied. For example, the likelihood of a diagnostic EEG is lower for older patients (37). More optimistic authors believe that with repeated EEGs, over 90 percent of patients with temporal lobe epilepsy may eventually admit of an EEG diagnosis, but three or more recordings, with sleep or other special procedures, may be needed (38).

Of all the EEG special procedures, all-night sleep deprivation probably is most productive. This procedure involves keeping the patient awake all night without stimulants, and then obtaining at least 90 minutes of EEG on the next day. In a recent French study (39), 22 patients with clinical diagnoses of partial epilepsy received EEGs before and after sleep deprivation. Before sleep deprivation, 27 percent had normal EEGs, but all showed abnormalities afterward. The occurrence of spike activity was 27 percent before and 59 percent after the activation procedure. Another European study showed that all-night sleep deprivation increased the yield of paroxysmal findings by 37.4 percent in a group of 88 patients with clinically diagnosed partial epilepsy (40). The technique of the second study required 3 to 5 hours of EEG recording on the day following sleep deprivation.

Because the psychiatrist without access to an epilepsy referral center will probably have to settle for less than comprehensive EEG investigation, the false negative rate will be higher. Pragmatically, then, a well-founded clinical suspicion of temporal lobe epilepsy should not be negated by normal or nonspecific EEG findings. Meticulous history-taking and interviews with witnesses to seizures are most helpful. As noted above, an EEG during or immediately following a typical seizure often can resolve a doubtful case.

IMPROVING THE FORMULATION OF THE NEUROLOGIC DIFFERENTIAL DIAGNOSIS

The formulation of a psychosocial diagnosis requires integration of information from the developmental history, the family history, and the clinical interview. The development of a useful and plausible neurologic differential diagnosis similarly requires an integration of diverse information from the history of present illness, the family history, the mental status examination, the neurological examination, and laboratory tests. Schizophrenia is not diagnosed from mental status findings alone, nor should mental status findings or laboratory tests be used in a simplistic way to categorize a case as organic or functional. It is more useful to generate for each case a plausible list of organic conditions that might be causal or contributory to the patient's mental disorder. Contributory problems are more common than causal problems and may be more often neglected because the nonorganic factors in the case may be of impressive magnitude.

We have found it a useful discipline to think in every psychiatric case of three plausible organic conditions the patient might have given their history, examination, and laboratory findings. The points below have been useful to us in formulating neurologic differential diagnoses for psychiatric patients.

Hard neurologic signs should never be dismissed as irrelevant. Borson (41) described a man recurrently treated for various "functional" psychiatric diagnoses while receiving a medical diagnosis of inactive Behcet's disease. Despite a deteriorating course with psychiatric symptoms accompanied at times by abnormal gait and rigid posture, the psychiatric disorder was not related by his physicians to Behcet's disease. This seems puzzling in view of the known involvement of the CNS by that disorder. Behcet's disease is a form of vasculitis which usually presents with oral and genital ulcers and recurrent ocular inflammation. CNS involvement, which may include meningoencephalitis, occurs in approximately 25 percent of patients (42). In another instance (43), a woman with coma induced by opiate overdose was misdiagnosed as hysterical because of apparent intermittent alertness and forcible eye closure when the examiner tried to open her eyes. Hard neurologic signs included hyperreflexia, difficulty swallowing, and coma vigil. The EEG was diffusely abnormal and the CT scan showed cerebral edema. Other cases have been reported of psychotic patients with cerebellar disease on CT scan, dysarthria, ataxia, and unilateral difficulty on tests of coordination who were diagnosed as functional (44), and of a subdural hematoma ultimately diagnosed by EEG and CT scan that presented with depression, ataxia, and fluctuating mental status with periods of relative alertness erroneously taken as evidence for a functional etiology (45).

Soft neurological signs and nonspecific psychiatric symptoms are most meaningful when occurring in combinations suggestive of specific diagnoses. Neurological signs and symptoms must be interpreted in a proper context. Repeated examinations and a search for independent confirmatory signs may be needed. Organic illnesses that are most frequently misdiagnosed include myasthenia gravis, hyperthyroidism, multiple sclerosis, normal pressure hydrocephalus, brain tumor, chronic subdural hematoma, and pancreatic carcinoma (46). Clues, although perhaps subtle, often exist, such as tremor with hyperthyroidism, gait disturbance with normal pressure hydrocephalus, and gait disturbance and headache with subdural hematoma.

There are a number of methods of seeking supporting evidence for suspected neurologic disease (47). These include 1) identifying mild facial asymmetry with the help of old photographs; 2) finding that rapid alternating movements are done more slowly in the dominant hand (the opposite is usually the case); 3) eliciting pathologic posturing of the hand, arm, or shoulder during gait tasks or mental status questions; and 4) finding *unilateral* occurrence of finger flexor reflexes such as the Hoffman sign, together with other motor abnormalities suggestive of neurologic disease. The Hoffman sign is elicited by holding the patient's hand palm downwards and resting the tip of the patient's middle finger on the examiner's index finger. Flicking the middle fingernail with the examiner's thumb evokes flexion of all the fingers on the abnormal side. The sign shows finger flexor reflexes are hyperactive, and is suggestive of pyramidal tract disease.

While unilateral signs usually are diagnostically meaningful, bilateral signs do not necessarily imply the presence of neurologic disease. Frontal release signs such as the snout reflex are found in a significant proportion of the normal population (48). Babinski signs are present after strenuous exercise in 7 percent of normal subjects (49, 50).

In patients with considerable abnormality of behavior, it may be impossible to perform the subtle sensory and visual field examinations that may be needed to identify parietal lobe lesions. In one reported case of parietal infarctions presenting psychiatrically, the onset of psychiatric illness in midlife coupled with a history of hypertension suggested the neurologic etiology (51).

The clinical diagnosis of multiple sclerosis often is based on a diagnostic history plus signs that, in themselves, would be nonspecific. Kellner et al. (52) reported two cases of patients hospitalized with rapid cycling bipolar illness who eventually were found to have multiple sclerosis. In the first instance, the patient had right-sided muscle spasms at 22 following an episode in her teens of visual disturbance. She had been earlier diagnosed as suffering a conversion reaction. The second patient developed a mood disorder at age 46 and at age 49 developed paresthesia and stiffness in her legs and poor coordination. At age 52, in light of a progressive gait disturbance, she received a lumbar puncture at which time oligoclonal bands were found in the CSF. Multiple sclerosis may be associated with unipolar or bipolar affective illness. A typical scenario would be presentation with "hysteria" and neurologic symptoms out of proportion to neurologic signs, followed after a variable period by harder neurologic findings. The combination of a vague intermittent neurologic history with affective disorder should lead a psychiatrist to consider multiple sclerosis. If bedside examination shows soft signs such as hyperactive reflexes and mild incoordination, multiple sclerosis should be pursued with particular vigor. In this situation, ancillary tests such as evoked potentials and special eye examinations are worthwhile.

Patients whose behavioral symptoms get worse on neuroleptics may have an undiagnosed organic disorder. Walker (53) cites three patients with organic disease (one with a left basal ganglia infarct and two with cortical atrophy) who experienced a deterioration of mental status on phenothiazines that was not reversed with antiparkinson drugs. Once a neuroleptic is given, significant neurological abnormalities may be attributed to the drug rather than to the possibility of underlying brain disease. The neurological assessment of the unmanageable catatonic patient, particularly in the emergency setting, is facilitated by administering diazepam rather than a neuroleptic (54). Neuroleptics may further confuse the clinical picture and cause a clinician to miss a treatable neurologic disease. The neuroleptic malignant syndrome may mimic catatonia. In this instance, diazepam would help whereas neuroleptics could worsen the condition.

Diagnostic exclusion of an organic basis for patient's symptoms is impossible early in a course of many illnesses. Psychiatric symptoms may be harbingers of organic illness—such as lupus, demyelinating disease (e.g., multiple sclerosis), degenerative brain disease (e.g., Huntington's chorea), and other illnesses—months to years before the emergence of hard neurological signs. Oommen et al. (55) reported on a case of Herpes Type II virus encephalitis that presented as a confusional psychosis without other neurologic signs with a normal CT scan and EEG. The CSF was positive and the diagnosis was confirmed at autopsy. Four other such cases were found in the literature. Clinicians cannot assume that viral encephalitis is not present because of the absence of hard neurologic signs and abnormal laboratory tests. Yik et al. (56) reported a recurrent psychiatric disorder (including exhibitionism) commencing in a woman at age 42 that was ultimately attributable to hepatic encephalopathy. The covert diagnosis of hepatic portal vein occlusion was made 5 years after the onset of psychiatric symptoms. Neurologic signs that waxed and waned were present but there were no peripheral stigmata of liver disease early in the course of the illness.

Depression with profound weight loss without a personal or family history of depression is suggestive of brain tumor, pancreatic carcinoma, a hormone-producing tumor, or endocrine cancer. Frontal and temporal cerebral metastases are particularly likely to present with psychiatric symptoms (57). In one study, 22 percent of patients with frontal tumors presented with psychiatric symptoms (58). Spinal cord tumors may be misdiagnosed as conversion disorders (59).

Peroutka (60) reported a case of a 72-year-old woman with the onset of auditory hallucinations and paranoid delusions due to a right temporoparietal-occipital lesion found on CT scan. Only an isolated neuropsychological test finding and a history of a focal seizure and reversible focal motor dysfunction pointed toward a neurologic disorder.

In lupus patients, 20 to 40 percent develop a psychiatric disorder such as delirium, dementia, or depression (61). EEG and CSF usually show abnormalities but occasionally are normal in definite cases. Neurologic signs pointing to an organic etiology for psychosis may appear some time after the presentation of schizophreniform psychoses in patients with numerous diseases of the basal ganglia and adjacent regions such as idiopathic calcification, Wilson's disease, Huntington's chorea, postencephalitic parkinsonism, bilateral subthalamic infarctions, and brain stem encephalitis (62). The absence of definite neurologic abnormality on initial screening does not permit the clinician to relax vigilance regarding the subsequent development of neurologic signs. Particularly in cases of Huntington's disease and Wilson's disease, diagnoses have been missed because the subsequent development of parkinsonism or involuntary movement was attributed to neuroleptics rather than considered as possibly indicating further evolution of an organic disease with psychiatric manifestations.

CONCLUSION

The identification of neurologic disease causing or contributing to psychiatric disorder would be greatly facilitated if psychiatrists would apply to neurologic assessment the same principles that are currently applied to psychodynamic assessment and formulation. First, no historical point or physical sign should be dismissed as irrelevant. Instead, efforts should be made to tie together various details to make a coherent and plausible picture. Second, both the neurological examination and laboratory tests should be seen as ways to test hypotheses developed from thinking about the patient's history. Infrequently used tests should be considered if they are known to be helpful in investigating a serious diagnostic possibility. If abnormalities are encountered, these should lead to the generation of new hypotheses to be tested by further investigations, therapeutic trials, or observation of the clinical course. Third, one must always remain an agnostic about the etiology of psychiatric symptoms. Just as an apparently organic patient may reveal a personal secret that explains much of the psychopathology, a patient with apparently functional illness may evolve blatant neurologic disease when observed over time. Avoiding premature closure and learning to enjoy the complexity and ambiguity of clinical situations is the psychiatrist's best defense against diagnostic error.

REFERENCES

1. Hall RCW, Popkin MK, Gardner ER, et al: Physical illness presenting as psychiatric disease. Arch Gen Psychiatry 35:1315–1320, 1978

2. Hall RCW, Gardner ER, Stickney S, et al: Physical illness manifesting as psychiatric disease. II. Analysis of a state hospital inpatient population. Arch Gen Psychiatry 37:989–995, 1980

3. Hall RCW, Gardner ER, Popkin MK, et al: Unrecognized physical illness prompting psychiatric admission: a prospective study. Am J Psychiatry 138:636–641, 1981

4. Koranyi EK: Morbidity and rate of undiagnosed physical illness in a psychiatric clinic population. Arch Gen Psychiatry 36:414–419, 1979

5. Tsuang MT, Woolson RF, Fleming JA: Premature deaths in schizophrenia and affective disorders: an analysis of survival curves and variables affecting the shortened survival. Arch Gen Psychiatry 37:979–983, 1980

6. Johnson DAW: The evaluation of routine physical examination in psychiatric cases. Practitioner 200:686–691, 1968

7. Slaby AE, Lieb J, Tancredi LR: The Handbook of Psychiatric Emergencies. 3rd ed. New York, Medical Examination Publishing Co, 1984

8. Brizer DA, Manning DW: Delirium induced by poisoning with anticholinergic agents. Am J Psychiatry 139:1343–1344, 1982

9. Epstein RS: Withdrawal symptoms from chronic use of low-dose barbiturates. Am J Psychiatry 137:107–108, 1980

10. Berlin RM, Conell LJ: Withdrawal symptoms after long-term treatment with therapeutic doses of flurazepam: a case report. Am J Psychiatry 140:488–490, 1983

11. Adler LE, Sadja L, Wilets G: Cimetidine toxicity manifested as paranoia and hallucinations. Am J Psychiatry 137:1112–1113, 1980

12. Shalmlan R: An overview of folic acid deficiency and psychiatric illness, in Folic Acid in Neurology, Psychiatry and Internal Medicine. Edited by Botez MI, Reynolds EH. New York, Raven Press, 1979

13. Caine ED, Shoalson I: Psychiatric syndromes in Huntington's disease. Am J Psychiatry 140:728–733, 1983

14. Rappolt RT, Gay GR, Farris RD: Emergency management of acute phencyclidine intoxication. Journal of the American College of Emergency Physicians 8:68–76, 1979

15. Ling MHM, Perry DJ, Tsuang MT: Side effects of corticosteroid therapy: psychiatric aspects. Arch Gen Psychiatry 38:471–477, 1981

16. Dubin WR, Weiss KJ, Zeccardi JA: Organic brain syndrome: a psychiatric imposter. JAMA, 249:60–62, 1983

17. Reulen JPH, Sanders EA, Hogenhuis LAH: Eye movement disorders in multiple sclerosis and optic neuritis. Brain 106:121–140, 1983

18. Guarino JR: Auscultatory percussion of the head. Br Med J [Clin Res] 284:1075–1077, 1982

19. Jenkyn LR, Walsh DB, Culver CM, et al: Clinical signs of diffuse cerebral dysfunction. J Neurol Neurosurg Psychiatry 40:956–966, 1977

20. Brizer DA, Manning DW: Delirium induced by poisoning with anticholinergic agents. Am J Psychiatry 139:1343–1344, 1982

21. Bass BJ: Acute mood and behavior disturbances of neurological origin: acute confusional states. J Neurosurg Nurs 14:61–68, 1982

22. Rimel RW, Tyson GW: The neurologic examination in patients with a central nervous system trauma. J Neruosurg Nurs 11:148–155, 1979

23. Levin HS, Madison CF, Bailey CB, et al: Mutism after closed-head injury. Arch Neurol 40:601–606, 1983

24. Kupersmith J, Nelson JI, Seiple WH, et al: The 20/20 eye in multiple sclerosis. Neurology 33:1015–1020, 1983

25. Sudarsky L, Ronthal M: Gait disorders among elderly patients. Arch Neurol 40:740–743, 1983

26. Robins PV: Reversible dementia in the misdiagnosis of dementia: a review. Hosp Community Psychiatry 34:830–835, 1983

27. Kiloh LG, McComas AJ, Osselton JW, et al: The values and limitations of electroencephalography, in Clinical Electroencephalography. 4th ed. Edited by Kiloh LG. London, Butterworths, 1981

28. Sotaniemi KA: Cerebral outcome after extracorporeal circulation. Arch Neurol 40:75–77, 1983

29. Evans DL, Edelson GA, Golden RN: Organic psychoses without anemia or spinal cord symptoms in patients with vitamin B12 deficiency. Am J Psychiatry 140:218–221, 1983

30. Griffith JF, Ch'ien LT: Herpes simplex virus encephalitis: diagnostic and treatment considerations. Med Clin North Am 67:991–1008, 1983

31. Nyback H, Wiesel FA, Berggren BM, et al: Computed tomography of the brain in patients with acute psychosis and in healthy volunteers. Acta Psychiatry Scand 65:403–414, 1982

32. Evans NJR: Cranial computerized tomography in clinical psychiatry: 100 consecutive cases. Compr Psychiatry 23:445–450, 1982

33. Fariello RG, Booker HE, Chun RW, et al: Reenactment of the triggering situations for the diagnosis of epilepsy. Neurology 33:878–884, 1983

34. Lesser RP, Lueders H, Conomy JP, et al: Sensory seizure mimicking a psychogenic seizure. Neurology 33:800–802, 1983

35. Ballenger CE, King DW, Gallagher BB: Partial complex status epilepticus. Neurology 33:1545–1552, 1983

36. Engel J, Driver MV, Falconer MA: Electrophysiological correlates of pathology and surgical results in temporal lobe epilepsy. Brain 98:129, 1975

37. Ajmone-Marsa C, Zivin LS: Factors related to the occurrence of typical paroxysmal abnormalities in the EEG records of epileptic patients. Epilepsia 11:361–381, 1970

38. Driver MV, McGillivray BB: Electroencephalography, in A Textbook of Epilepsy, 2nd ed. Edited by Laidlaw J, Richens A. New York, Churchill Livingstone, 1982

39. Arne-bes MC, Calvet U, Thiberge M, Arbus L: Effects of sleep deprivation in an EEG study of epileptics, in Sleep and Epilepsy. Edited by Sterman MB, Shouse MN, Passouant P. New York, Academic Press, 1982

40. Declerck AC, Sijben-Kiggen R, Wauquier A, Marten W: Diagnosis of epilepsy with the aid of sleeping methodology: evaluation of 1,163 cases, in Sleep and Epilepsy. Edited by Sterman MB, Shouse MN, Passouant P. New York, Academic Press, 1982

41. Borson S: Behcet's disease as a psychiatric disorder: a case report. Am J Psychiatry 139:1348–1349, 1982

42. Petersdorf RG, Adams RD, Braunwald E, Isselbacher KJ, Martin JB, Wilson JD. (eds): Harrison's Principles of Internal Medicine. 10th ed. New York, McGraw-Hill, 1983

43. Shraberg D, D'Souza T: Coma vigil masquerading as psychiatric diagnosis. J Clin Psychiatry 43:375–376, 1982

44. Hamilton NG, Frick RB, Takahashi T, et al: Psychiatric symptoms in cerebellar pathology. Am J Psychiatry 140:1322–1326, 1983

45. Alarcon RD, Thweatt RW: A case of subdural hematoma mimicking severe depression with conversion-like symptoms. Am J Psychiatry 140:1360–1361, 1983

46. Martin MJ: Brief review of organic diseases masquerading as functional illness. Hosp Community Psychiatry 34:328–332, 1983

47. Massey EW, Scherokman B: Soft neurologic signs. Postgrad Med 70:66–67, 1981

48. Jacobs L, Glassman MD: Three primitive reflexes in normal adults. Neurology 30:184–188, 1980

49. Farrell MJ: Influence of locomotion on the plantar reflex in normal and physically and mentally inferior persons. Arch Neurol 46:222–230, 1941

50. Elliot TR, Walsh FM: The Babinski or extensor form of plantar response in toxic states, apart from organic disease of the pyramidal tract or systems. Lancet 1:65–68, 1925

51. Tippin J, Dunner FJ: Biparietal infarction in a patient with catatonia. Am J Psychiatry 138:1386–1387, 1981

52. Kellner CHR, Davenport Y, Post RM, et al: Rapidly cycling bipolar disorder in mutliple sclerosis. Am J Psychiatry 141:112–113, 1983

53. Walker WR: Phenothiazine therapy in latent organic brain syndrome. Psychosomatics 23:962–968, 1982

54. McEvoy JP, Lohr JB: Diazepam for catatonia. Am J Psychiatry 141:284–285, 1984

55. Oommen AJ, Johnson PC, Ray CG: Herpes simplex type II virus encephalitis presenting as psychosis. Am J Med 73:445–448, 1982

56. Yik KY, Sullivan SN, Troster M: Neuropsychiatric disturbance due to occult occlusion of the parietal vein. Can Med Assoc J 126:50–52, 1982

57. Peterson LG, Perl M: Psychiatric presentations of cancer. Psychosomatics 23:601–604, 1982

58. Strauss I, Keshner M: Mental symptoms in cases of tumor of the frontal lobe. Archives of Neurology and Psychiatry 33:986–1005, 1935

59. Epstein BS, Epstein JA, Postel DM, et al: Tumors of the spinal cord simulating psychiatric disorders. Diseases of the Nervous System 32:741–743, 1971

60. Peroutka SJ: Hallucinations and delusions following a right temporo-parietal occipital infarction. Johns Hopkins Medical Journal 151:181–184, 1982

61. Bresnahan B: CNS lupus. Clin Rheum Dis 8:183–195, 1982

62. Cummings JL, Gosenfeld LF, Houlihan JP, et al: Neuropsychiatric disturbances associated with the ideopathic calcification of the basal ganglia. Biol Psychiatry 18:591–601, 1983

Chapter 3

Psychiatric Manifestations and Implications of Seizure Disorders

Robert M. Post, M.D.
Thomas W. Uhde, M.D.
Russell T. Joffe, M.D.
Linda Bierer, M.D.

Chapter 3

Psychiatric Manifestations and Implications of Seizure Disorders

I n the early literature on the relationship of psychiatric illness to seizure disorders, contradictions were apparent. Jackson (1) described the different psychiatric manifestations of preictal, ictal, and interictal states. He suggested that there was a close interrelationship between seizures and psychological phenomena and that the definition of epilepsy be expanded to include some mental aberrations:

> I think, as I have elsewhere suggested, that the term [epilepsy] should be degraded to stand for our knowledge, or rather for our ignorance of the various permanent and temporary conditions of nerve tissue in functional divisions, or perhaps in nutritive regions, which conditions cause or prevent temporary failures or losses of functions. Thus epilepsy would not, in this sense, convey the idea of convulsions, but of temporary disorders of functions of many kinds, sensory as well as motor and mental as well as physical. (p. 328)

In contrast, others have emphasized the possible reciprocal relationships between seizures and psychosis (2, 3), observations that indirectly led to the introduction of convulsive seizures, or electroconvulsive therapy (ECT), as a therapy for psychiatric illness and the current refinement of ECT as a major effective treatment modality for manic and depressive episodes. Thus, on the one hand, there were keen observers of behavior who noted many psychiatric abnormalities occurring with and as a result of various types of seizures; on the other, major motor seizures were induced as a therapeutic modality.

The controversies that have abounded about the nature of psychiatric disturbances occurring in epileptics continue to the present day. In this chapter we will attempt to elucidate some of the variables that account for this obviously complex set of relationships, both positive and negative, between seizures and psychiatric disturbances. Some investigators have suggested that there are characteristic

35

interictal personality changes in patients with complex partial seizures (4–7), whereas others argue against this proposition (8–13). In this chapter we will focus on the complexities of the relationship of major psychiatric disturbances to seizures with the hope that some of the important variables may be pertinent to the on-going controversy regarding more subtle personality disturbances. See Table 1 for the evidence marshaled by Stevens (8) to support the argument for lack of differences.

Elucidating some of the variables involved in the differential effects of seizure disorders on major psychiatric manifestations may help to fulfill the promise that understanding seizure disorders may be an important step toward understanding the neurobiology of psychiatric disorders. Just as Freud postulated that the interpretation of dreams was the "royal road to the unconscious," many neurologists have suggested that the pathological firing of epileptic neurons might provide important road maps to the normal connectivity and functioning of the nervous system involved in both neurological and behavioral disorders.

At present, another epoch in the interrelationship of psychiatric disorders and seizure disorders is unfolding. In addition to ECT as a therapeutic modality, some anticonvulsant compounds used in the treatment of seizure disorders are now increasingly recognized as useful treatments for manic-depressive illness (14, 15). While the early claims for phenytoin have not yet been supported by systematic and double-blind clinical trials, controlled investigations have indicated that carbamazepine, valproic acid, and clonazepam may have useful antimanic effects. In addition, there are indications that carbamazepine may have acute antidepressant effects and a considerable body of evidence indicates that carbamazepine may be useful in the prophylactic treatment of manic-depressive illness (15–19). These data will be briefly reviewed and discussed from the theoretical perspective that common treatments for seizures and psychiatric disorders imply at least some common pathophysiological mechanisms.

PSYCHIATRIC MANIFESTATIONS OF COMPLEX PARTIAL SEIZURES

Major Psychiatric Syndromes

Psychosis. The series of Gibbs (20) and Slater et al. (21) provided numerical support for the long-appreciated clinical observations that patients presenting with psychomotor seizures (temporal lobe epilepsy, complex partial seizures) might be prone to the development of interictal psychoses, which at times could mimic those observed during schizophrenic syndromes. Gibbs reported on 678 patients with psychomotor epilepsy and 1,800 with psychomotor and grand mal epilepsy from an original cohort of 10,000 patients. Forty percent of the patients with temporal lobe epilepsy (TLE) and 50 percent of the patients with TLE plus grand mal seizures had some psychopathology compared with 10 percent for the other seizure types. A large literature has now accumulated attempting not only to describe the incidence and clinical characteristics of the psychoses associated with complex partial seizures, but also to define possible predictors or risk factors for this form of decompensation.

These risk factors have been reviewed by Stevens (8) and include deep or diffuse structural (or physiological) brain abnormalities, abnormal neurological examination, postchildhood onset of seizures, central nervous system infection, and reduced psychomotor seizure frequency (Table 2). In addition, Hermann et al. (22) reported that an aura of ictal fear was a predictor of more severe psychiatric disturbances in epileptics. These data are of interest in relationship to the findings of Gloor et al. (23) that fear was produced by stimulation of deep limbic structures (i.e., amygdala) and not the overlying neocortex. If the aura of intense fear reflects involvement of limbic structures, this relationship of fear to subsequent psychiatric disturbance could suggest that activation of these limbic pathways is an important determinant of later psychiatric difficulties. Flor-Henry (24), Dongier (25), and Kristensen and Sindrup (26) have found psychosis to be inversely correlated with the frequency of psychomotor–psychosensory seizures in patients with TLE. Thus the presence of a seizure disorder may increase the possibility of psychiatric disturbances, but in some instances, in the face of this increased relationship, the occurrence of seizures themselves and psychopathology may vary inversely.

Although the psychotic episodes of patients suffering from psychomotor seizures have been described by many as "schizophreniform," a wide variety of clinical presentations has also been reported. As illustrated in Table 3, affective illness, anxiety disorders, and confusional syndromes may also be prominent. These major psychiatric disturbances associated with epilepsy often appear to mimic those found in the primary psychiatric disorders. The parallels have been confirmed by Perez and Trimble (27) using modern classificatory schemas. Although the psychosis of TLE may characteristically include inappropriate or bizarre behavior, paranoid and religious delusions, and hallucinations "typical" of schizophrenic decompensations, Glaser (28) and Perez and Trimble have noted a continued effort to remain in social contact and a lack of autism or of archaic

Table 1. Psychological Testing of Matched Epilepsy and Control Populations

Investigators	Subjects	Examination	Generalized Versus TLE
Matthews and Klove (154)	44 TLE 52 major motor 98 brain-damaged 51 normals	MMPI	No differences
Mignone et al. (36)	98 TLE 53 non-TLE	MMPI	No differences
Glass and Mattson (155)	40 TLE 13 generalized 13 focal/non-TLE	MMPI	No differences
Standage and Fenton (156)	19 TLE 18 non-TLE	Present State Examination (Wing)	No differences

Hermann et al. (22)	47 TLE 28 non-TLE	MMPI	No differences
Rodin et al. (157)	A. 56 TLE only B. 22 TLE and generalized C. 46 non-TLE (1 seizure type) D. 32 non-TLE and other	WAIS, MMPI	A. Better WAIS, MMPI than B, C, and D B. More paranoid personality, psychosis, and job problems than A, C, and D C. More organic signs, job difficulty, anticonvulsants than D

Note. Table compiled by Stevens (8). TLE = temporal lobe epilepsy. MMPI = Minnesota Multiphasic Personality Inventory. WAIS = Wechsler Adult Intelligence Scale.

or personalized thinking that may differentiate these episodes from those of schizophrenia. A prominent affective component (29, 30) is frequently present during these psychotic episodes.

Affective Disorder. Robertson and Trimble (31) have also studied depressive episodes in epileptics, but direct diagnostic comparisons with primary depression using Research Diagnostic Criteria (RDC) (31a) or the *Diagnostic and Statistical Manual of Mental Disorders,* Third Edition (DSM-III) (31b) have not, to our knowledge, been employed. While melancholia has been reported as the most common interictal disturbance in epileptic patients admitted for psychiatric care, anxiety and fear are more frequently reported as an ictal effect (32–34). Robertson (35) reported that 40 percent of her patients showed an endogenous pattern of depression, but that depressive psychosis was rare. Depression was also characterized by high anxiety, neuroticism, hostility, and feelings of depersonalization; these characteristics were not influenced by age of onset, type of epilepsy, or laterality of focus (although left side was slightly overrepresented in the seizure frequency). Robertson and Trimble noted that in other studies (36, 37), depression was common in those with late onset

Table 2. Risk Factors for Psychopathology in Patients with Epilepsy

	A (%)	B (%)	A/B
Psychomotor epilepsy	30.6	30.2	1.0
TLE	30.0	30.0	1.0
TLE (MMPI)	22.0	30.0	0.73
Age of onset 9 years[a]	22.3	5.0	4.5
Sphenoid spikes[b]	21.0	5.0	4.2
Multiple spikes[b]	22.7	6.0	3.8
Automatism or visceral aural[b]	11.4	6.4	1.8
Abnormal neurological examination	21.0	8.3	2.5
Psychomotor seizure frequency 1/week[a]	6.1	11.6	0.525
History of febrile seizures[a]	6.0	9.5	0.63
Family history of epilepsy[a]	5.2	10.6	0.49

Note. From Stevens (8). A = Number of patients with psychosis, psychiatric hospitalizations, or other severe psychopathology (PS) with risk factors (RF), divided by total PS with RF; B = Number with PS without RF, divided by total PS without RF; A/B = Increase or decrease of PS in risk with each RF.

[a]From Kristensen and Sindrup (26). Arbitrary incidence of psychosis: 10%.

[b]From Taylor (158). Arbitrary incidence of schizophrenia-like psychosis: 10%.

Table 3. Incidence of Affective Illness in Psychiatrically Ill Patients with Temporal Lobe Epilepsy

Investigators	N	Affective Illness		Schizophreniform		Confusional Syndromes		Anxiety Disorders		Other	
		N	%	N	%	N	%	N	%	N	%
Dalby (39)	54	20	37	4	7					30	56
Dongier (25)	236	70	30	49	21	117	50				
Mulder and Daly (49)	62	16	26	20	32			36	58	4	6
(14 duplications)											
Flor-Henry (41)	50	9	18	21	42	9	18			11	22
Perez and Trimble (27)	16	2 or 5	13 or 31	11	69						
Currie et al. (50)	40	4	10	12	30			7	18	17	43
Pritchard et al. (93)	20	2 or 7	10 or 35	3	15					16	80
(6 duplications)											
Shukla et al. (159)	49	5	10	11	22	1	2	6	12	26	53
Small et al. (160)	44	2	5	6	6	14	32	6	14	16	36
Parnas et al. (161)	25	1	4	3	12					21	84
Total	596	139	23	140	23	141	24	55	9	141	24

seizures. They also reviewed a series of studies indicating a 4- to 5-times greater incidence of suicide in epileptics compared to that expected in a normal population and a 25-time greater risk in those with TLE.

The relative rarity of manic syndromes in epilepsy has been observed (38–40), although Flor-Henry (41) and Dongier (25) reported substantial seizures with manic-depressive or manic diagnoses. Careful longitudinal analysis of a large series of patients, using modern diagnostic criteria, would appear to be indicated.

Anxiety and Panic Syndromes. Harper and Roth (42) discussed the close parallels between cases of TLE and phobic anxiety-depersonalization syndromes. They have suggested that

> Incomplete investigation of certain abruptly developing disturbances of behavior and consciousness, particularly in a setting of acute and erroneous anxiety, may often lead to diagnosis of epilepsy. . . . It is suggested that the location in the temporal lobes of controlling mechanisms concerned with arousal and anxiety may account for the resemblances between the two types of illnesses. (p. 221)

Jackson (43) observed that "it is not uncommon for a patient to have the emotions of terror and to look terrified at the outset of his seizures." Fear is among the most common ictal emotions, usually occurring with visceral sensations (44). Among 2,000 unselected patients, Williams (34) observed fear in 61 of 100 patients with ictal emotions. Fear as an aura is usually of brief duration, but longer and recurring bouts of intense anxiety have been described in cases of complex partial seizure status epilepticus with complete resolution of the anxiety and ictal fear following temporal lobectomy (45, 46). Stimulation of the temporal cortex with fiber connections to the amygdala is thought to be the final common pathway for the elicitation of the illusion of fear (23, 47). Heath et al. (48) reported a patient who experienced intense fear with an impulse to run developing on repeated stimulation of the amygdala with depth electrodes after initial stimulations were associated with rage reactions.

Although the reported percentages differ, several investigators have noted that anxiety states are prominently represented among the interictal manifestations of TLE. In their early study of 100 non-institutionalized patients with electroencephalogram (EEG) evidence of temporal lobe foci whose presenting complaints were initially diagnosed as psychiatric, Mulder and Daly (49) found that 36 patients complained of anxiety, irritability, somatic manifestations, and dissociative episodes. These symptoms, that in this series antedated the diagnosis of psychomotor seizures, are typical of the presenting complaints of patients with panic anxiety disorders. Indeed, in a series of 666 patients with TLE, Currie et al. (50) found evidence of interictal anxiety in 19 percent of their sample, and noted that anxiety or depression antedated the first clinical manifestations of a seizure disorder in 48 (7 percent) patients.

Several features of panic attacks are strikingly similar to those reported by a substantial minority of patients with TLE who experience fear or anxiety as a preictal aura. Williams (34) studied 165 patients with "complex feelings" as part of their epileptic attacks; 100 were noted to experience ictal emotions. Of these, 61 patients reported ictal fear, with 21 patients reporting feelings of depression during attacks. Daly (44) found 25 of 52 temporal lobe epileptics reported ictal fear with another 14 patients reporting feelings of anxiety and other unpleasant sensations they felt were akin to fear. Penfield quoted his patients' referring to their ictal emotions with the words: "fear, loneliness, sadness, scared feeling, terror" (51, p. 458). As these emotions are frequently accompanied by vasomotor or visceral disturbances that also accompany the experience of panic anxiety (42, 44), several investigators have examined the differential presentations and long-term consequences of these two disorders.

In a classic study, Harper and Roth (42) compared in detail the presentations and histories of 30 patients with panic anxiety syndrome to 30 patients with TLE. Although episodic anxiety was experienced significantly more frequently by patients with panic anxiety disorders, 53 percent of their seizure disorder patients also reported episodic anxiety attacks. Episodic disturbances of speech and automatic behaviors were significantly more prevalent in patients with TLE, but motor or sensory visceral changes did not distinguish between the groups. While derealization and jamais vu experiences were significantly more prevalent in the patients with panic anxiety disorder, depersonalization, hallucinatory and illusory experiences, perceptual distortions, and the idea of "a presence" were common to both disorders. Unlike the attacks of temporal lobe epileptics that tended to end as abruptly as they began, panic attacks tended to terminate gradually.

The differential diagnosis of panic anxiety and psychomotor seizure disorders, especially in the early stages of TLE, may depend on the use of techniques designed to elicit EEG evidence of epileptiform activity. Brodsky et al. (52) described 10 patients, originally diagnosed as "borderline state" or "latent schizophrenia," who suffered from "attacks of anxiety" (sometimes accompanied by impulsive behavior) and who were unresponsive to various psychotropic medications and demonstrated "paradoxical" reactions to neuroleptics. With 24-hour sleep-deprived EEGs, temporal lobe abnormalities were revealed in each that had not been evident with routine EEG examination. Although this study is intriguing, it must be remembered that the diagnosis of TLE is a clinical one and does not rest on characteristic EEG findings in isolation.

The interictal manifestations of patients with psychomotor seizures who experience ictal fear may differ from those in whom, although an aura may be present, fear is not experienced. Hermann et al. (22) have examined a sample of 11 temporal lobe epileptics with ictal fear as a prominent sign, matched with 11 similar patients with gustatory or olfactory auras, and compared to 14 patients with generalized seizure disorders. Minnesota Multiphasic Personality Inventory (MMPI) profiles revealed significantly more psychopathology in the ictal fear group when compared with both the temporal lobe nonfear and generalized seizure disorder groups. Scores for the Psychopathic deviate, Paranoia, Psychasthenia, and Schizophrenia subscales were all elevated in the patients experiencing ictal fear. In addition, 45 percent of the patients with ictal fear, only 7 percent of the temporal lobe patients without ictal fear, and none of the generalized seizure disorder patients had been admitted to a psychiatric hospital. These data suggest that ictal fear may identify a subgroup of patients with TLE with a differential vulnerability to the development of interictal psychopathology.

Identification, therefore, of the neuroanatomic substrate(s) involved in the expression of fear may provide a clue to the pathophysiology of the behavioral disturbances that develop in patients experiencing this symptom as an ictal aura. In 1955, Heath et al. (48) published a case report of a "schizophrenic" patient in whom feelings of "unreality" had led to the progressive development of anxiety, estrangement, and agoraphobia. Stimulating electrodes were implanted in the region of the amygdaloid nucleus of this patient, who initially reported a feeling of rage when electrically stimulated, but whose response rapidly changed to one of intense fear on subsequent stimulations. Gloor et al. (23) reported a similar case of a patient whose ictal manifestations included a sense of fear accompanied by palpitations. Stimulation of various regions of the temporal lobe with depth electrodes during a neurological procedure was undertaken. Discharge confined to the hippocampus did not elicit a subjective response, but as soon as the discharge involved the amygdala, the patient reported feeling "scared." Stimulation of the amygdala directly produced this feeling of fear. Henriksen (45) reported the coincidence of EEG evidence of almost continuous spike activity in the sphenoidal leads with the experience of anxiety in a patient whose psychomotor fits were successfully treated by anterior temporal lobectomy that included the basolateral amygdala. These cases illustrate in humans what has been repeatedly described as fearful or defensive attack behaviors elicited by amygdaloid stimulation in animal models (53–55).

The report of Belluzzi and Grossman (56) of the development of a deficit in avoidance learning in rats in whom seizures have been produced by microinjection into the amygdaloid complex serves to implicate further the amygdala in the development of long-lasting behavioral pathology. Moreover, the behaviors elicited in animals and those reported in human studies are remarkably convergent. Amygdaloid stimulation leads to the expression of fearful and aggressive behaviors in animals and of similar affects in humans. The potential development of both learned helplessness and chronic aggression in animal models is analogous to the development in humans of avoidant behaviors and of violent discontrol (57), which have been suggested to be delayed consequences of pathological discharge in this nucleus. An understanding of the neurobiology and pathophysiology of the amygdala and of the amygdala-hippocampal circuit may be particularly relevant, then, to the study of several of the psychopathological features of patients with TLE.

Psychiatric Correlates of the Laterality of Seizure Focus

The question has been repeatedly raised of an association between the side of the temporal focus and the nature of the psychotic disturbance seen in psychomotor epilepsy. In 1969, Flor-Henry (24, 41) reviewed a series of 50 temporal lobe epileptics with documented histories of psychosis and suggested that patients with left temporal lobe foci might be prone to psychotic episodes with a schizophreniform appearance compared to those with right-sided foci, who tended to show manic and depressive syndromes.

Sherwin (58) has recently reviewed these findings and presented his own data, which suggest that epileptic patients with schizophreniform psychoses may be overly represented among those with left compared with right temporal lobe foci. Among this series of 61 patients with unilateral temporal lobe lesions who underwent surgical lobectomy, only 4 percent of the 46 patients with right-sided lesions had histories of psychosis, whereas 33 percent of the 15 patients with left-sided lesions evidenced such a history. These psychoses were characterized by Sherwin as "schizophrenia-like." Support for this association was provided by the developmental study of Lindsay et al. (59) who prospectively followed 89 children with TLE and found that of the 10 percent who developed "schizophreniform" psychoses, none had right-sided lesions, 7 had left-sided lesions, and 2 were bilateral. The fact that Flor-Henry (41) reported no differences in the incidence of psychosis in patients with bilateral when compared with unilateral left-sided (but not right-sided) lesions is worth noting. He suggested that involvement of the left temporal lobe, whether or not the right side is also involved, is the critical variable in the development of this form of psychosis.

Trimble (60) has summarized much of the literature suggestive of a predominance of left-sided temporal lobe lesions in patients with a schizophrenic-like psychosis (Table 4). Kristensen and Sindrup (26), however, have reported no laterality differences in 96 psychomotor seizure patients with paranoid hallucinatory psychoses compared to 96 patients without this psychiatric disturbance. Bruens (61) suggested that more extensive and multifocal epileptic illness was more likely to be associated with psychosis; for example, while he found a 6 percent incidence of psychosis in patients with pure generalized or pure psychomotor seizures, he observed a 33 percent incidence of psychosis in patients with the combination.

The literature appears ambiguous regarding the association of right temporal lobe foci to affective disorders. While case reports have suggested an association of mania with a right-sided focus (62), investigations of the relationship of depression to focus laterality have produced varied results. Robertson and Trimble (31) reported a slightly increased incidence of left-sided foci in their patients with TLE and depression. Small et al. (63) reported that six manic patients

Table 4. Left- and Right-Sided Temporal Lesions in Patients with a Schizophreniform Psychosis of Epilepsy

Investigators	N	Left	Right	Bilateral
Slater et al. (21)	48	16	12	20
Flor-Henry (41)	21	9	2	10
Gregoriadis et al. (162)	43	43	0	0
Taylor (75)	13	9	4	0
Hara et al. (163)	10	6	4	0
Sherwin (72)	6	5	1	0
Sherwin (58)	7	5	2	0
Toone et al. (164)	12	4	0	8
Ounsted and Lindsay (165)	9	7	0	2
Trimble and Perez (65)	11	8	2	1
Total	180	112	27	41
		(62.2%)	(15.0%)	(22.7%)

Note. From Trimble (60).

undergoing right unilateral ECT uniformly deteriorated, but responded well to bilateral ECT, suggestinig the possible involvement of the untreated left hemisphere in their mania.

In a carefully diagnosed and lateralized series, Perini and Mendius (64) found that patients with left compared to right hemisphere of seizure onset monitored by closed-circuit television-EEG telemetry showed significantly higher levels of depression on the Beck Depression Inventory and the Spielberger Trait Anxiety Scale. It must be remembered, however, that Flor-Henry (41) sampled patients with psychosis and his assertions pertain to patients whose psychiatric presentations resembled those of the major psychotic disorders.

Studies of the interictal personality or character traits of temporal lobe epileptics, in which the laterality of the discharge focus was also known and investigated, have provided some interesting and related findings. Trimble and Perez (65) compared Present State Examination symptom profiles of patients with left- and right-sided temporal lobe foci separated by EEG criteria. Left-sided patients showed significantly increased scores for "nuclear schizophrenia" and ideas of reference when compared to right-sided patients. Using an 18-item symptom scale developed to assess traits that have been associated with temporal lobe epileptics, Bear and Fedio (5) reported that right temporal lobe epileptics reported significantly more elation and tended to "polish" their self-image compared to observer reports, whereas left-sided patients reported significantly increased paranoia and dependence and tended to "tarnish" their self-reports. In a psychological investigation of right- versus left-sided temporal lobe epileptics, McIntyre et al. (66) reported an atypical reflective response style of patients with left-sided pathology in which they made idiosyncratic interpretations of verbal representations of affective states and a style characterized by impulsivity for patients with right-sided lesions. Forrest (40) reported on a rapid cycling manic-depressive syndrome occurring in an epileptic who had had his right hemisphere surgically removed; this case, although complicated by early brain damage and epilepsy, suggests that the left hemisphere and remaining brain tissue are sufficient to produce syndromes highly similar to manic-depressive illness.

In a study of 36 patients, Serafetinides (67) found an increased incidence of aggression in the 25 patients with left-sided EEG abnormalities compared with the 11 patients with right-sided EEG abnormalities. Flor-Henry (41) reported orgasmic epilepsy was associated with a right-sided form, and Sackeim et al. (68) indicated that gelastic (laughing attack) seizures were exclusively right-sided. Kolb and Taylor (69) found that patients with temporal, parietal, or frontal lobe lesions showed impaired appreciation of affect on a visual task (matching different faces displaying similar emotional states), whereas those with left-sided lesions showed impaired matching of verbal descriptions of emotional states. These data are consistent with a large literature regarding hemispheral specialization of emotional functions and suggest the potential importance of lateralization of seizure focus in the development of secondary psychiatric disturbances.

Reciprocal Relationships Between Seizures and Psychosis

The complexity of the relationships between complex partial seizures and depression is further emphasized by the findings of Engel et al. (70) at UCLA. They have not only observed a high incidence of depressive disorders among their patients with complex partial seizures (71), but they also noted a substantial incidence of severe depression occurring for months to years following successful treatment of complex partial seizures by removal of the temporal lobe focus. These data again highlight possible reciprocal relationships between seizures and major psychiatric syndromes. In this instance, the control of seizures achieved by surgical removal of the focus appeared to be a predisposing factor toward the development of severe endogenous depression. Parallel observations have been reported by Sherwin (72), Stevens (73), Jensen and Larsen (74), and Taylor (75) with the development of schizophreniform psychoses following successful treatment of seizures with temporal lobectomy. Stevens reported that of 14 patients operated on between 1956 and 1970, 11 became seizure free; 8 of these 11 had no prior psychiatric history, yet 3 of these 8 developed disabling paranoid psychosis. Jensen and Larsen observed psychosis in 6 of 45 epileptics who achieved good seizure control following temporal lobectomy.

These data are consistent with the considerable literature suggesting the reciprocal relationship between seizures and psychosis (2, 24, 25, 76–78). Landolt (2) observed the phenomenon of "forced normalization," that is, the EEG became more than usually well organized in association with the development of severe behavioral pathology. Others have observed the onset of major psychiatric difficulties with the achievement of anticonvulsant control of seizure disorders (77).

Specificity of Psychiatric Manifestations

The association of both affective syndromes and schizophrenia-like syndromes with complex partial seizures (Table 2) raises the issue of the specificity of psychiatric syndromes that may occur with TLE.

Stevens (8) and others have argued that psychiatric manifestations are generally no more common in patients with complex partial seizures than they are with other types of seizure disorders and perhaps in other neurological illnesses. Stevens has emphasized that patient selection factors may bias the results reported in the literature. Stevens notes that complex partial seizures represent up to 80 percent of seizure disorders, such that a patient presenting with psychiatric difficulties who is subsequently found to have a seizure disorder would be more likely to have complex partial seizures than other seizure types. Therefore, Stevens believes that a relationship between complex partial seizures and other psychiatric manifestations has been overestimated in the literature. Yet Alving (79) reported that all 21 of 1,500 epileptics with schizophrenic-like psychosis had complex partial seizures whereas none of 276 patients with primary generalized seizures was schizophrenic.

The study of Dongier (25) may be particularly informative in relation to the issue of seizure type and the specificity of associated psychiatric symptomatology. As summarized in Table 5, patients' symptomatology was classified as confusional, affective, or schizophreniform. There were no substantial differences in the distribution of psychiatric correlates of different seizure types. While confusion was significantly more likely to occur with centrencephalic seizures, patients with frontal lobe seizures appeared to have a roughly similar distribution of these psychiatric syndromes as compared to those with temporal lobe seizures. These data suggest both the potential nonspecificity of the type of psychiatric symptomatology associated with a single epileptiform disorder or one in various brain areas. These data are important because of the large number of patients studied, but also require replication and clarification in light of modern diagnostic classificatory schemas, as well as several caveats. It is possible, even in some focal seizures, that disordered neural circuitry is involved at some distance from the epileptiform focus, and that temporal lobe and limbic substrates may be affected in patients with generalized seizure disorders, as well as in patients with more selective involvement of these areas. Nonetheless, preliminary conclusions from this study would suggest that considerable caution should be exercised in assuming a direct relationship between seizure type and psychiatric manifestation.

The need for caution regarding specificity is further supported by the data summarized in Table 6, where a partial list based on a selective review of the literature is presented on the many different psychiatric manifestations that have been reported in patients with complex partial seizures. Presumably, a more comprehensive review would

Table 5. Interictal Psychoses and Type of Epilepsy

	Centren-cephalic		Temporal Lobe		Frontal Lobe		Others		Total	
	N	%	N	%	N	%	N	%	N	%
Confusional	138	64	117	50	11	52	33	52	299	56
Affective	50	23	70	30	8	38	15	23	143	27
Schizophreniform	27	13	49	21	2	10	16	25	94	18
Total	215	40	236	44	21	4	64	12	536	100

reveal even more syndromes and better documentation. Nonetheless, the current list suffices to make the point that a myriad of psychiatric presentations have been associated with complex partial seizures. These include not only typical syndromes such as affective and schizophreniform psychoses, but also a variety of isolated psychiatric symptoms such as gelastic attacks and more elaborate types of psychopathology, such as multiple personality syndrome.

Table 6. Diverse Psychiatric Manifestations Associated with Temporal Lobe Epilepsy

Syndrome or Symptom	Selected References Investigators
Affective Psychosis	Dongier (25); Dalby (39); Flor-Henry (41)
Schizophreniform Psychosis	Slater et al. (21); Kristensen and Sindrup (26); Stevens (166); Sherwin (58); Taylor (75)
Panic Anxiety	Gloor et al. (23); McLachlan and Blume (46); Currie et al. (50); Harper and Roth (42)
Personality Changes	Bear and Fedio (5); Bear et al. (7)
Aggression	Serafetinides (67); Ashford et al. (167); Ramani and Gumnit (76); Rodin (168); Delgado-Escueta et al. (169)
Ecstatic Seizures (Dostoevsky Epilepsy)	Cirignotta et al. (170)
Demonic Possession	Mesulam (171)
Religiosity	Waxman and Geshwind (4)
Suicidality	Pritchard et al. (93)
Sexual (Orgasmic)	Flor-Henry (172); Mandell (173); Heath (174)
Gelastic	Sackeim et al. (68)
Multiple Personality Syndrome	Mesulam (171); Schenk and Bear (175)
Transient Global Amnesia	Tharp (176)
Cognitive Perceptual Alteration (Psychosensory Symptoms)	Dalby (113); Penfield (177); Gloor et al. (23)
Depersonalization (Mental Diplopia)	Jackson and Stewart (178)

Assuming that many of these observations and case reports do represent the association of diverse psychiatric symptoms with complex partial seizures in excess of what might be expected in neurologically normal populations, what inferences might we draw from this great variety of psychiatric symptomatology? What variables might help determine the type of symptomatology observed? The study by Engel et al. (70) of regional glucose metabolism, utilizing positron emission tomography (PET) scan techniques with 2-deoxyglucose, is particularly informative in this regard. In a series of patients with complex partial seizures, Engel et al. found that there was a large variety of patterns of increased glucose utilization observed during ictal periods, even in patients presenting with relatively similar types of seizure manifestations. Moreover, repeat studies of the same patient during more than one seizure indicated that the pattern of glucose utilization might differ from seizure to seizure within the same individual. Thus some of the apparent nonspecificity of behavioral and psychiatric correlates of seizure disorders may be derived from the fact that different pathways are involved in seizures classified under the broad category of "complex partial" or "psychomotor" epilepsy. The potential variability within a given individual's neural circuitry obviously adds further to the difficulties of interpretation.

Moreover, in patients studied interictally, there were decreases in glucose utilization in the same brain regions that had previously been activated when studied during the ictus. Thus a variety of interictal psychopathology may be related either to the brief, periodic, intense activation of neural circuits associated with increased firing during the seizure and associated increases in glucose utilization, or with the interictal appearance of significantly decreased metabolic activity. These data are also of interest in relation to the suggestion reviewed above that anxiety may be a more common ictal than interictal affect, whereas depression may be a more prominent interictal emotion.

These data are also consistent with those of Trimble (60) who reported decreases in glucose utilization among epileptic patients presenting with psychotic disorders. These PET data again emphasize the potential importance of the relationship of behavioral pathology to preictal, ictal, postictal, or interictal neural changes. In addition, Gale et al. (71) reported that EEG evidence for the side of the epileptic focus did not always correspond to that observed on PET scan and that the PET localization appeared to be more accurate and to yield better postoperative results following temporal lobe resection. This might further account for some of the controversies regarding laterality of lesion and psychiatric symptomatology discussed above.

ANIMAL MODELS FOR SEIZURES AND PSYCHOPATHOLOGY

Environmental Context of Seizures and Behavioral Change

A variety of physiological and psychological considerations may be particularly important in considering the ultimate behavioral correlates of seizure disorders. Valenstein (80), Kopa et al. (81), and Belenkov and Shalkovskaya (82) have all emphasized that the behavioral consequences of electrical stimulation of a given area of brain may differ considerably according to environmental contingencies and behavioral state. For example, Kopa et al. demonstrated that a cat given stimulation of the thalamus when it was on a platform previously associated with nonshock or food reward produced positive affective reactions, while stimulation of the same area of brain with the same parameters in an environment previously associated with shock or punishment produced a very different and negative affective reaction. If these consistent observations of the importance of environmental context and behavioral state on type of response produced are extrapolated to the clinical situation, we might surmise that a whole host of clinical, environmental, and psychological variables applicable at the time of the ictus are highly relevant to the ultimate development of behavioral pathology.

An early case of Penfield and Rasmussen (83) is illustrative of a related phenomenon that experiences may influence ictal process and content. A 14-year-old female patient with temporal lobe seizures incorporated the content and affect of a fearful experience into the hallucinations accompanying her seizures. At age 7, she had been approached by a man who asked her if she wanted to get into a bag of snakes he was carrying. The episode, which was witnessed by her brothers, was reexperienced during her psychomotor seizures. The seizures became so intractable that surgery was recommended and performed. Under local anesthesia, stimulation of points on the exposed occipital or temporal cortex could selectively reproduce the appropriate visual or auditory "hallucinations" of the experience as well as the associated feelings of dread and terror.

The memory of this early event appeared to be encoded in a facilitated pathway that could be reactivated 1) in dreams; 2) in the epileptiform discharges of her psychomotor seizures; 3) with specific cortical stimulation; or more interestingly 4) with conscious recall. Once the temporal lobe area involved in the initial pathological discharge was surgically removed, the patient no longer experienced seizures or the hallucinations of the episode but could still consciously recall the experience when she "voluntarily summoned the memory," suggesting that the memory might also have been coded in the opposite temporal lobe, which was not involved in the seizure discharges. We emphasize in this example that critical emotional and cognitive experiences have the potential for being encoded and facilitated in such a way that they may erupt into awareness (without conscious recall) in a dream, in a hallucination, or on direct cortical stimulation and that this facilitatory or memory-like process is represented with some anatomical and physiological specificity and redundancy. Thus it would also appear that individual idiosyncratic, psychologically and psychodynamically relevant issues may be differentially incorporated into different components of the seizure, as well as being encoded in associated circuitry that can survive extirpation of the pathological temporal lobe focus.

The Valenstein (80) effect represents another and important variation on this theme. These investigators reported that hypothalamic stimulation produced differential behavioral effects, depending on the availability of food or water. Most notably, in either instance, repeated stimulation of the same area of the hypothalamus with the same current characteristics began to elicit increasingly greater food or water intake, depending on which was available.

These laboratory and clinical data highlight both the importance of the environmental context for associated behavioral manifestations connected with stimulation of a given neural pathway and the possibility that repeated stimulation of this pathway (even with precisely the same current characteristics) may be associated with progressive increases in the behavioral consequences.

Kindling and Its Behavioral Consequences

This focus on the longitudinal development of behavioral pathology in relation to repeated stimulation over time of the same neural pathways deserves considerable emphasis. The phenomenon of kindling may offer an experimental model with which to explore the neurophysiologic basis of this relationship. In electrophysiological kindling, a given area of brain is repeatedly and intermittently stimulated with a given current. This stimulation is associated with a lowering of the threshold for afterdischarges that begin to emerge with increasing duration and complexity, and spread to other areas of the brain beyond those originally stimulated. Eventually, the animals will develop a major motor seizure following a repetition of stimulation that was previously subthreshold. In addition, if these kindled seizures are repeated with sufficient frequency, a phase of "spontaneity" will ensue where the animal develops seizures in the absence of exogenous electrophysiological stimulation.

These observations, originally described by Goddard et al. (84) and named "kindling" in 1969, have now been well demonstrated and replicated in many laboratories and are summarized in Table 7. These data may be relevant from several perspectives. They may provide a useful model not only for the longitudinal development of seizure disorders themselves, but of their associated behavioral concomitants. In terms of seizure kindling, some patients with irritative foci might not develop overt seizures until many repetitions of paroxysmal firing in a given pathway. This model might help explain the "ripening" effect described by Penfield and other neu-

Table 7. Major Characteristics of Electrical Kindling

---

1. Repeated stimulations
   a. Initially subseizure threshold
   b. Intermittent

2. Local afterdischarges and seizure activity
   a. Increases in amplitude, frequency
   b. Increase in duration
   c. Increase in complexity of wave form
   d. Increase in anatomical spread

3. Replicable sequence of seizure stages
   Behavioral arrest, blinking and masticatory movements, head nodding, opsithotonis, contralateral then bilateral forelimb, clonus, rearing, and falling

4. Discharges kindle in quantum jumps

5. Limbic system kindles more readily than cortex

6. In kindled animals the history of convulsion development is recapitulated as seizure builds

7. Transfer effects to secondary sites; kindling facilitated in other sites even after primary site destroyed

8. Interference: A secondary kindled site interferes with primary site rekindling

9. No toxic or neuropathological changes evident; kindling is a transsynaptic process

10. Relatively permanent change in connectivity; a kindled animal will still seize after a 1-year seizure-free interval

11. Seizure may develop spontaneously in chronically kindled animals

12. Interictal spikes and spontaneous epileptiform potentials develop

---

Note. See Goddard et al. (84) regarding 1, 4–10; Wada and Sato (179) regarding 2–4, 6; Wada et al. (180) regarding 10–12; Racine (181); and Pinel and Rovner (182, 183).

rologists in conceptualizing the long lag period and delay between initial trauma or onset of a given lesion and the onset of seizure disorder (83). The data are also interesting from the perspective of spontaneity. During the phase of spontaneous seizures, an electro-physiological reorganization appears to take place. The spontaneous seizure is no longer associated with an afterdischarge at the original kindled focus in the cortex (85). These data may be relevant in considering some patients with apparent "hysterical" seizures where seizure behaviors are evident but the EEG evidence of an underlying focus is not manifest.

During the kindling process, there is an obvious progression of increasing neurophysiological and behavioral reaction to a given stimulation over time. Not only does the afterdischarge grow and spread to other areas of the brain, but the behavioral manifestations of seizures go through a sequential series of stages from behavioral arrest (stage 1); to head nodding, chewing, and whisker twitching (stage 2); to unilateral forepaw extension and seizure clonus (stage 3), to bilateral seizure involvement of forepaws as well as the head and trunk (stage 4); to rearing and falling (stage 5).

We may ask whether a parallel set of progressive phenomena may not occur for behavioral impairments not directly associated with the seizure process. For example, in the Valenstein (80) effect, increasing food and water intake is apparent with successive stimulations of the same area of brain. Following repeated *subconvulsive* administration of lidocaine (which itself can produce a kindled seizure), a progressive development of bizarre ingestive behaviors is observed where animals increasingly mouth and eat inedible objects (86). Adamec (87) has emphasized that repeated amygdala stimulation below that sufficient to produce overt seizures can change the personality of laboratory cats in a long-lasting fashion. This pre-kindling stimulation is sufficient to produce a lowered afterdischarge threshold. Concomitant with this change in excitability of the amygdala, he observed long-lasting alterations in the animals' placidity and aggressive behavior. Adamec observed that cats that were spontaneous killers of rats had significantly higher amygdala afterdischarge thresholds than nonkiller animals. When these killer cats were kindled to lower their amygdala afterdischarge threshold (increase amygdala excitability), they became nonkillers. Thus repeated activation of a given set of neural circuits could not only alter the threshold and setpoints for excitability of those circuits, thus altering the associated behavioral consequences in a long-lasting fashion, but may, in some instances, produce progressive increases in behavioral pathology with repeated (even subconvulsive) stimulation.

In 1976 we first postulated that a kindling mechanism might be pertinent not only to seizure development in epilepsy, but also to some of the associated behavioral alterations (88, 89). Repeated activation of temporal lobe and limbic substrates could ultimately produce seizures and abnormalities in associated pathways critical for the regulation of emotional and cognitive function. We suggested that such a kindling-like process could result in behavioral alterations as a result of dysfunction or disconnection in a given pathway, based on the observation that an excitatory focus can produce greater behavioral impairments than ablative lesions in experimental animals (90). Bear (6) extended and modified this model, suggesting that a kindling process would lead to sensory-limbic "hyperconnection" that in turn would contribute to the development of behavioral pathology. In support of this hypothesis, Bear et al. (91) reported that patients with TLE showed more responsive skin conductance changes to emotional and neutral photographic stimuli. However, Bellur et al. (13) have suggested that this may have been due to an enhanced orienting response rather than increased emotional responsivity because the increased electrodermal response also occurred to neutral stimuli. Moreover, using controls with seizures not involving temporal lobes, Bellur et al. did not find evidence of increased autonomic responsiveness to visual stimulation in the temporal lobe epileptics.

If behavioral disorders are "kindled" in parallel with or as a result of seizure development, then the onset of these behavioral disturbances might be expected to follow the onset of the seizure disorder. Some support for this postulate is provided in Table 8, summarizing recent literature on the lag between seizure onset and the development of behavioral pathology. In these studies, the average lag of a decade or more between the first seizure and the development of psychopathology is at least not inconsistent with a kindling process. However, a more convincing demonstration would be that the lag would be independent of the age of onset of seizure disorder, that is, those with late onset seizures should have an equally long lag before the development of psychopathology and a comparatively later age of onset of psychiatric difficulties. This relationship was confirmed by Slater and Moran (92) for females, but not males. However, data of Pritchard et al. (93) in children suggest that psychopathology develops at about the same time, in early adolescence, regardless of the age of seizure onset (Figure 1). In addition, Stevens (8) has pointed out the similarity in age of onset of psychosis in epileptics to that observed in uncomplicated schizophrenia, suggesting that similar predisposing variables (not the epilepsy) may be important.

The distributions of age of onset of TLE and affective illness appear relatively similar (Figure 2), so that a demonstration of a similar lag of a decade between onsets of TLE and affective illness might suggest a pathophysiological connection.

The production of seizures in given areas of the brain using the kindling process in animals provides a controlled means for exploring some of the variables involved in the production of behavioral con-

Table 8. Interval Between Onset of Seizures and Psychosis

	N	Age Onset Seizure	Age Onset Psychosis	Interval
Yde et al. (184)	20	45	29	−16
	7	13	25	12
Gastaut (185)	83	20.6	31.7	11
Serafetinides and Falconer (186)	12	14.5	27	12.5
Slater et al. (21)	69	15.7	29.8	14.1
Slater and Moran (92)				
M		19.3	34	14.8
F		12	25.2	13.2
Glaser (28)	37			6
Jus (187)	15			13
Flor-Henry (41)	50	13	24	11
Bruens (188)	19	13	25	12
Standage (189)	5	15.6	34.7	19.1
Trixler and Nador (190)	7			14
Kristensen and Sindrup (26)	96	21	34	13
Peters (191)	8	13.4	26.9	13.5
Sugano and Miyasaka (192)	21	14.8	28	13.2
Ramani and Gumnit (193)	10	10.8	16.4	5.6
	N = 439	mean = 15	27.8	11.8
				(weighted mean interval)
				12.1
				(unweighted mean interval)

comitants of seizures. These might include pathway stimulated; age of onset; frequency, intensity, and spread of activity; ongoing personality; environmental variables; genetic predisposition; and other variables of clinical import.

A variety of behavioral disturbances have been associated with kindling or related types of repeated stimulation of the brain (Table 9). For example, we observed that repeated stimulation of the amygdala sufficient to result in amygdala-kindled seizures produced a long-lasting decrement in spontaneous exploratory hyperactivity and in cocaine-induced exploratory activity. Ehlers et al. (94) replicated and extended these findings with the observation that amphetamine-induced hyperactivity was reduced following kindled seizures not only of the amygdala but also of the nucleus accumbens. Although Pinel et al. (95) reported that repeated kindled seizures of the amygdala and hippocampus, but not of the caudate nucleus, were associated with increases in aggression and irritability, Bawden and Racine (96) and workers in our laboratory have not replicated these findings.

Pharmacological Kindling

We have observed that repeated seizures induced with the local anesthetic lidocaine are associated with the onset of irritability and

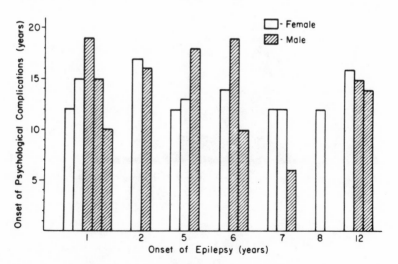

Figure 1. Age at Onset of Temporal Lobe Epilepsy Versus Age at Appearance of Psychological Complications

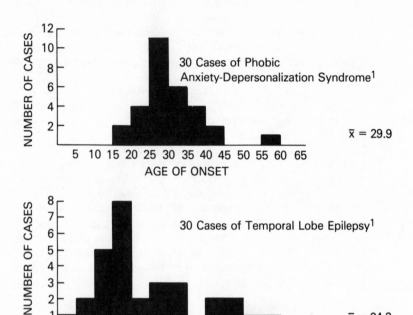

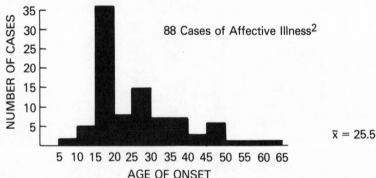

[1]From Harper & Roth, 1962
[2]Post, Unpubl. Data, 1983

Figure 2. Age Distributions of the Phobic Anxiety-Depersonalization Syndrome, Temporal Lobe Epilepsy, and Affective Illness

Table 9. Behavioral Effects of Electrical Kindling: Long-Lasting Spontaneous and Drug-Induced Alterations

Effect	Investigators
Amygdala kindling	
Decreased rat killing (cat)	Adamec (87)
Decreased spontaneous rearing and decreased cocaine-induced rearing (rat)	Post et al. (194)
Decreased amphetamine-induced hyperactivity (rat)	Ehlers et al. (94)
Decreased exploration[a] (rat)	Weingartner and White (195)
Weight gain (rat)	Innes et al. (196)
Increased aggression (rat) (not replicated)	Pinel et al. (95) Bawden and Racine (96)
Increased predatory response (rat)	McIntyre (197)
Increased rage reaction[a] (cat)	Yoshi and Yamaguchi (198) Gunne and Reis (199)
Increased play, decreases and increases in aggression[a] (monkey)	Deflorida and Delgado (200)
Inhibitory avoidance (rat)	Boast and McIntyre (201)
Decreased conditioned emotional response (reversed by adrenalectomy in rat)	McIntyre (197) McIntyre and Molino (202)
Intense fear (humans)	Heath et al. (203)
Mood change and pressure of speech[a] (human)	Ervin et al. (204) Stevens et al. (205) Goddard and Morrell (206)
Nucleus accumbens kindling	
Decreased amphetamine-induced hyperactivity (rat)	Ehlers et al. (94)
Hippocampal kindling	
Increased aggression (rat)	Pinel et al. (95)
Lateralized state-dependent learning (rat)	Stokes and McIntyre (207)
Ventral tegmentum (A10) kindling	
Increased bizarre behavior and decreased social activity (cat)	Stevens and Livermore (208)
Hypothalamus kindling	
Increase in food intake[a] (cat)	Delgado and Anand (209)
Increase in food or water intake (rat)	Valenstein et al. (210)
Lower eating and drinking thresholds[a] (rat)	Wise (211)

[a] Not typical kindling paradigm.

aggression, particularly directed toward laboratory personnel who handle the animals. Weiss et al. (97) have demonstrated that intra-cerebroventricular administration of the neuropeptide corticotropin-releasing factor (CRF) (which produces behavioral and EEG seizures similar to those achieved following amygdala kindling) also produces marked changes in irritability and aggression (in this case, independent of whether the animals demonstrate seizures). The CRF-induced irritability and aggression appear to be more predominantly directed toward conspecifics (other rats) rather than toward laboratory caretakers on handling of the animals.

Although further work is required to delineate the mechanisms involved in the late onset of seizures and aggressive behavior following intracerebroventricular administration of CRF, these findings are of potential clinical import. They suggest the possibility that endogenously secreted neuropeptides may, under some conditions, be associated with alterations in neural excitability sufficient to produce seizures or irritable and aggressive behavior. The fact that CRF is a major hormonal mediator of the stress response (fight or flight) in animals and presumably also in humans and may also be involved in depressive disorders (98) may ultimately yield important insights regarding the possible relationships of stressful environmental events to subsequent development of psychiatric and ictal pathology.

The long-lasting changes in irritability and aggression observed following the experience of lidocaine-kindled seizures illustrates an additional point. While there has been considerable debate in the clinical literature on the relationship of complex partial seizures and aggression, particularly whether aggressive acts are committed during the ictus, our data would suggest the utility of also examining the interictal period and considering the long-term consequences of having had a temporal lobe seizure. That is, there may be clinically relevant alterations in the thresholds or predispositions for aggressive behavior in patients long after they have ceased to experience ictal manifestations. This is particularly apparent in the lidocaine-kindled seizure model; during the ictus and immediately in the postictal period, these animals are not irritable and aggressive but become so in the interictal period (99). Because these seizures are intimately associated with brain structures involved in cognitive processing, learning, and memory, one might also address the issue in animals of whether this altered behavioral responsivity is based on disturbed cognition. Data of Mellanby (100) are partially consistent with this formulation. In her model of tetanus toxin-induced limbic seizures, learning deficits and aggression were reversed by carbamazepine in some instances, even when seizures were not inhibited.

The long-lasting consequences for aggressive behavior and the long-lasting changes in locomotor activity, observed following kindling of the amygdala and nucleus accumbens in laboratory rats (Table 9), support the proposition that there may be important consequences for human behavior following a series of complex partial seizures. Although it is obviously tenuous to generalize from the animal laboratory to human psychopathology, we suggest the usefulness of these animal models to uncover relevant variables that may be of importance in the study of epileptic patients and may account for the variability in their associated psychiatric symptomatology (Tables 3 and 6).

Cocaine Seizures and Panic Attacks: A Kindling-Like Mechanism?

We and others have demonstrated that repeated administration of the same dose of the local anesthetic cocaine to rats, cats, dogs, and monkeys not only produces behavioral sensitization (increased behavioral pathology) to a variety of endpoints, but may, under appropriate circumstances, result in the production of seizures following a dose of drug that had previously been subconvulsant (101). Repeated administration of low doses of cocaine leads to increased motor responsivity to cocaine in the rat. The mechanisms underlying this behavioral sensitization effect are not known but are thought to relate to the drug's psychomotor stimulant (probably dopaminergic) properties and to involve a robust environmental context or conditioning component (102, 103). These data indicate that (like the context-dependent effect of electrical stimulation reviewed above) similar psychological and conditional variables may influence the degree of behavioral responsivity to psychomotor stimulants and, potentially, to other stressors as well (103).

Based on our experience with the pure local anesthetic lidocaine (99), we believe that the local anesthetic components of cocaine may, in a similar fashion, be sufficient to produce a pharmacological kindling effect. The sensitization and kindling data may be particularly important to the growing epidemic of human cocaine abuse and its associated behavioral and convulsive toxicity. Increasingly high doses of cocaine are being self-administered by many routes, including oral, intranasal (snorting), intravenous, and inhaling coke paste (free basing). Very high blood levels of cocaine can be achieved with any of these modes of administration and when cocaine is used in a repeated fashion it can parallel the procedures utilized in the laboratory to produce pharmacological kindling.

In a series of 500 patients interviewed by Washton and Gold (104), a 17 percent incidence of blackouts and seizures was reported. Although a variety of factors may account for the development of cocaine-related seizures in a substantial percentage of cocaine users (including variable purity and doses of cocaine), a kindling process might provide one explanation for the apparent emergence of seizures to doses that had been previously administered and found to be subconvulsive for a given individual. Moreover, since tolerance may develop to the euphorogenic properties of cocaine, this may lead some users to administer increasingly high doses to achieve or sustain peak mood elevation. Thus repeated bouts of extremely high doses of cocaine may be produced that either in themselves are sufficient to produce seizures or, because of a kindling-like process, ultimately lead to seizures from a dose that ordinarily would be subconvulsive. When Deneau et al. (105) allowed rhesus primates free access to cocaine, they repeatedly administered cocaine in sufficient quantities to produce seizures and ultimately death.

Moreover, our findings with repeated administration of local anesthetics in laboratory animals, indicating that progressive alterations in behavior may be observed in the absence of seizure production, also raise the possibility that some of the psychiatric side effects of local anesthetic administration could be occurring in a kindling- or sensitization-like fashion (99). The potential implications of the chronic administration of cocaine for alterations in affective states and the emergence of paranoid–schizophreniform-like psychoses are discussed elsewhere (106).

In this chapter we would like to emphasize one other psychiatric syndrome developing from repeated cocaine administration. Uhde and associates (unpublished observations, 1984) have noted a group of patients entering their clinic for the study of panic and anxiety disorders who reported the onset of their panic attacks occurring with cocaine administration. One of these cases is illustrated in Figure 3. This was a 26-year-old man who described a 3-year history of essentially daily cocaine administration by the intranasal route without notable anxiety symptoms. However, in January 1974 he noted the onset of a severe anxiety reaction that reached panic proportions shortly after the administration of intranasal cocaine. Over the next 6 months he continued to have panic attacks approximately 5 times a week following cocaine administration. The panic attacks were not experienced each time after cocaine administration, which continued on a daily basis, but when they did occur, they immediately followed the use of cocaine. After approximately 100 of these cocaine-related panic attacks, in July 1974 he developed his first panic attack in the absence of cocaine administration. (It is of considerable interest that hundreds of amygdala-kindled seizures are required before an animal

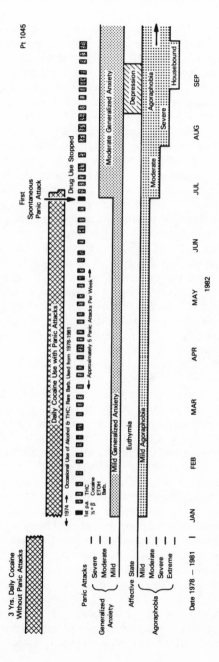

Figure 3. Development of Panic Disorder Following Cocaine Use

achieves spontaneous seizures, perhaps paralleling the 100 cocaine-related panics achieved by this patient prior to his first spontaneous panic attack.) Shortly following this panic attack, the patient ceased using cocaine and yet continued to demonstrate repeated spontaneous panic attacks. These were subsequently treated with alprazolam, carbamazepine, and imipramine, each with moderate to substantial success.

Washton and Gold (104) reported that approximately 50 percent of the first 500 callers on their recently established cocaine hotline gave histories of cocaine-induced panic attacks. These data and those of Washton and Tatarsky (107), also reporting a high incidence of panic attacks in cocaine users, together with the unpublished observations of Uhde et al. (as illustrated in Figure 3) suggest the possibility that a high proportion of cocaine abusers may, on a kindling-like sensitization basis, become increasingly prone to developing panic attacks and, if given sufficient repetitions, these may in some instances lead to the development of spontaneous panic disorder. Based on our work with the local anesthetic procaine (discussed below), which produces selective activation of fast EEG frequencies over the temporal cortex in humans (Coppola et al., unpublished manuscript, 1984), we would also suggest the importance of temporal lobe and limbic system structures in the development of this type of panic disorder.

Alcohol Withdrawal Syndromes and Kindling

Another complex neuropsychiatric syndrome that may be better understood from the kindling perspective is recurrent alcohol withdrawal and its concomitant neuropsychiatric and physiological concomitants. Alcohol is a potent anticonvulsant and, during its withdrawal, the brain goes through periods of increased neural excitability. We postulated (108, 109) that repeated episodes of this increased excitability associated with withdrawal of alcohol might be a sufficient stimulus to produce a kindling-like sensitization. We postulated that this could account for the ultimate development of alcohol withdrawal seizures in some individuals and could account for some of the sequential development of increasingly severe alcohol withdrawal symptomatology, progressing from shakes to increases in autonomic instability to full-blown delirium tremens. In addition to the convulsive and neuropsychiatric syndromes emerging during the acute withdrawal period, it is also of interest that a spectrum of psychiatric disorders appears to emerge as a late consequence of chronic alcohol administration, including alcoholic halucinosis, various personality changes, and psychiatric syndromes. Recently, it has also been recognized that alcoholics may suffer a high incidence of panic attacks (110), findings that are of interest in relationship to the postulated kindling mechanism discussed above (Figure 3). These observations also highlight the potential relationship between anxiety symptoms and a variety of convulsant mechanisms, including endogenous and exogenous electrical stimulations, as well as chemically induced changes.

Additional laboratory evidence now supports a kindling hypothesis for alcohol withdrawal (111), and one of the theoretical derivatives of the hypothesis—that anticonvulsants such as carbamazepine should be effective treatments of alcohol withdrawal syndromes—has received preliminary support (112).

ANTICONVULSANTS: EFFICACY IN AFFECTIVE DISORDERS

Carbamazepine in Primary and Secondary Affective Syndromes

One reason for initiating clinical trials of the anticonvulsant carbamazepine in patients with primary affective illness was the observation that this drug was effective in treating affective disturbances of patients with primary seizure disorders (39, 113). Dalby (113) indicated that many of the patients treated with carbamazepine for their epilepsy had improvement in associated dysfunction of mood and behavior. In particular, many epileptic patients with recurrent depressive illness showed greater improvement in their mood disorder than in their seizures. That is, some patients who showed inadequate seizure control had an excellent acute and prophylactic antidepressant response to carbamazepine. We were also impressed that carbamazepine was a particularly effective drug for dampening seizures thought to arise from limbic system substrates in both laboratory animal models (114–117) and clinical populations (118, 119). In addition, open clinical trials of carbamazepine in affectively ill patients suggested efficacy in patients without seizure disorders (120, 121).

Our current data and those of other investigators suggest that carbamazepine may possess acute antimanic and antidepressant effects as well as longer-term prophylactic efficacy in preventing manic and depressive recurrences (15, 18, 19, 122). Our patients were intensively investigated and studied to rule out a possible seizure disorder. Thus it appears that patients with affective disorders secondary to complex partial seizures, as well as those with primary affective illness without evidence of seizure disorders, are responsive to the anticonvulsant carbamazepine.

The efficacy of this anticonvulsant compound in both primary and secondary affective disorders, as well as in complex partial seizures and trigeminal neuralgia, raises several issues of clinical and theoretical import. Are the positive psychotropic effects of carbamazepine in affective illness related to the same biochemical and physiological effects of the drug that mediate its anticonvulsant efficacy? If this proves to be the case, are the properties responsible for carbamazepine's particular efficacy in limbic system disorders (as opposed to other areas of brain) also the ones that mediate its psychotropic effect?

As yet, we do not have definitive answers to either of these questions, but several lines of evidence bear on these questions and will be reviewed. Certainly, one must entertain the possibility that carbamazepine, with its panoply of biochemical and physiological effects on a variety of neurotransmitter, neuromodulator, neuropeptide substances (18, 123), could exert one series of effects that are important to its anticonvulsant properties and another set of effects that are important to its psychotropic effects. The fact that many potent psychotropic substances such as tricyclic antidepressants, neuroleptics, and lithium carbonate are effective in various phases of manic-depressive illness and are not potent anticonvulsants suggests the possibility that differential mechanisms of carbamazepine's action could account for its anticonvulsant and psychotropic properties. If such a dissociation did account for carbamazepine actions, it would be difficult to assess directly. Moreover, we are not aware of analogues of carbamazepine that exhibit such dissociated effects. In particular, three congeners—carbamazepine itself, its 10,11-epoxide metabolite, and a keto derivative of carbamazepine—are all potent anticonvulsants and all appear to also have important effects either in trigeminal neuralgia or in manic-depressive illness. Thus, at least with the carbamazepine moiety, it may be that the anticonvulsant, antinociceptive, and psychotropic effects are inextricably interwoven.

Even if it were the case that the carbamazepine's anticonvulsant effects did relate to its psychotropic properties, it would not imply that a seizure disorder necessarily underlies primary affective illness. In particular, carbamazepine is effective in patients with trigeminal neuralgia and related paroxysmal pain syndromes, which do not appear to involve a classic ictal process. Thus it is possible that neuronal dysregulation, including altered changes in excitability and paroxysmal discharges that do not involve an ictal process, could be common to a variety of neuropsychiatric syndromes and account for the effects of carbamazepine. The drug does have an interesting profile of clinical efficacy in syndromes that involve paroxysmal dysregulation of neural activity, including epilepsy, pain, motor phenomena, and affect.

Limbic Effects of Carbamazepine in Affective Illness

What lines of evidence bear on the question of whether carbamazepine's psychotropic properties are related to its proclivity to dampen limbic system excitability and limbic system seizures? One approach to this problem would be the demonstration that the rank order of drugs that are effective in inhibiting complex partial seizures in humans and in inhibiting limbic system seizures in experimental models would parallel the rank order of efficacy of anticonvulsants in treating manic-depressive illness. As illustrated in Table 10 from the review of Porter and Penry (119), carbamazepine emerged as one of the treatments of choice for complex partial seizures (118, 124, 125). Other effective agents included phenytoin, valproic acid, and clonazepam. There is some parallelism in the rank order of this listing derived from clinical studies and evidence from the studies of Albright and Burnham (117) regarding the ability of anticonvulsants to suppress limbic system foci (afterdischarges in the amygdala) compared to afterdischarges kindled from the cerebral cortex. Again, carbamazepine emerged as the drug with the greatest relative efficacy on amygdala versus cortical kindled seizures. Valproic acid was next and clonazepam was somewhat lower on the hierarchical list. These clinical and experimental animal model data are of interest in relation to the findings that, in addition to carbamazepine, valproic acid and clonazepam have been demonstrated in blind studies to show acute antimanic properties. Valproic acid and its congeners may also exert

Table 10. Results of Clinical Trials: Complex Partial Seizures

Drug	Number of Clinical Trials		
	Unchanged	Moderate	Excellent
Carbamazepine	—	1	8
Clonazepam	3	6	5
Valproate	2	5	3
Phenytoin	—	—	1
Primidone	—	1	1
Phenacemide	1	1	1
Methsuximide	2	4	—
Mephenytoin	—	2	—
Trimethadione	—	1	—
Paramethadione	1	—	—
Ethotoin	1	—	—
Metharbital	1	—	—
Phenobarbital	(No clinical trials)		

Note. From Porter and Penry (119).

long-term efficacy in the prophylactic management of patients with affective disorders, particularly when used in combination with lithium carbonate (126–131).

The studies with phenytoin require replication and extension. The early uncontrolled trials in the 1940s demonstrated mixed results. While Kalinowsky and Putnam (132) and Kubanek and Rowell (133) suggested that phenytoin might have useful effects in manic-depressive illness, this was not supported by the study of Freyhan (134), although he did report one patient with recurrent excited manifestations of apparently a schizoaffective process who did improve with the institution of phenytoin on four separate occasions and who deteriorated each time the drug was withdrawn. These data raise the possibility that some patients may respond to the anticonvulsant phenytoin, although the broader claims of Dreyfus (135) of the efficacy of this drug in a variety of neuropsychiatric syndromes remain to be demonstrated in controlled, systematic trials.

Although there is some evidence that the anticonvulsants that are relatively high on the clinical and experimental rank ordering for efficacy in complex partial and limbic system seizures show efficacy in manic-depressive illness, there is an absence of studies indicating that agents that are on the lower end of the rank ordering for limbic anticonvulsant effects, such as those used for the treatment of petit mal, are not efficacious in affective syndromes. Thus clinical trials of these different classes of anticonvulsants would be of theoretical import even if all the drugs were not effective in the treatment of manic-depressive illness. Assessing the differential biochemical and physiological effects of these agents might yield important information regarding their mechanisms of action in affective illness.

Data on specific limbic system dysfunction that might be affected by carbamazepine are also relatively lacking at this time. Yet preliminary evidence from PET scan techniques suggests that glucose utilization is not increased in temporal lobe and limbic system substrates in patients with affective disorders as it is in patients during complex partial seizures. In fact, data of Phelps (136) indicated decreased cortical glucose utilization in bipolar depressed patients compared to manic patients or normal controls. Recent data in our laboratory (in association with M. Buchsbaum, L. DeLisi, and R. Cohen) also suggest that depressed patients may have significantly decreased temporal lobe glucose utilization compared to schizophrenics and normal controls. Our series of patients who have had PET studies, followed by a clinical trial of carbamazepine, is not yet sufficiently large to answer the question of whether relative alterations in temporal lobe metabolic activity are related to subsequent clinical response to carbamazepine.

Similarly, we have tried to address the issue of whether clinical indicators of limbic system dysfunction are correlated with subsequent clinical response to carbamazepine. In collaboration with E. Silberman, we have assessed the degree that patients with primary affective illness have symptoms that have been closely associated with those observed in patients with psychomotor seizure disorder. J. Ballenger and others in our clinical research unit had observed many patients with profound sensory and cognitive alterations during their affective episodes. We developed a rating scale (the Silberman-Post Psychomotor-Psychosensory Inventory) and found that patients with affective illness did have significantly greater numbers of psychosensory symptoms than did a medically ill hypertensive inpatient comparison group (137, 138). Surprisingly, the total number of symptoms reported by patients with affective illness was similar to that reported by patients with complex partial seizures, although there were differences in the distributions of specific items (Figure 4). Interestingly, the occurrence of these symptoms was closely associated with episodes of mania or depression and not with the well

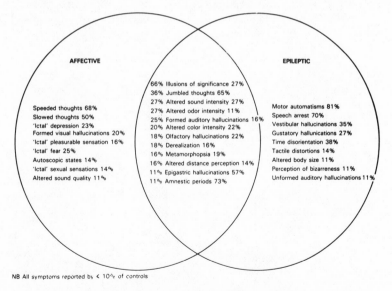

NB All symptoms reported by < 10% of controls

Figure 4. Distribution of Symptoms Reported by Patients with Affective Illness Compared with Patients with Epilepsy

interval (Figure 5). We had hypothesized that the occurrence of these symptoms might be an indirect marker for dysfunction in temporal lobe and limbic substrates, and, as such, might predict subsequent response to carbamazepine. On the contrary, we observed that an increased number of these psychomotor-psychosensory symptoms appeared to be associated with better clinical response to lithium carbonate (Figure 6) and, although the data are not yet complete, preliminary evidence suggests that this is not the case for carbamazepine.

It is particularly pertinent in this volume entitled *Medical Mimics of Psychiatric Disorders* to emphasize the fact that many psychiatric symptoms can mimic those found in neurological disorders without implying the same etiology. This appears to be a particularly important issue as some investigators (139) have used the presence of psychomotor-psychosensory symptoms to help make the diagnosis of seizure disorder. At this time, this would appear unwarranted in light of the emerging data that not only do a high percentage of patients with primary affective illness display these symptoms, but also many patients with panic anxiety disorder (140) and many patients with borderline personality disorder (R. Cowdry, personal communication, 1984) also show a high incidence of these symptoms. The work of Chapman (141) also suggests that many schizophrenic patients show a high incidence of these symptoms. Thus

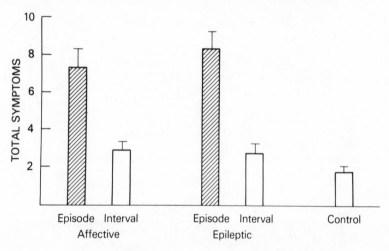

Figure 5. Mean Numbers of Symptoms Reported During Episodes of Illness Versus Internal Periods

it is possible that the presence of these psychomotor-psychosensory symptoms does, in fact, represent an index of dysfunction in temporal lobe and limbic system substrates. If this were the case, these symptoms would not appear diagnostically specific. The important question remains to be answered as to whether the patients with high numbers of these symptoms can be differentiated from other patients on the basis of other markers of limbic system dysfunction or differential treatment response.

A final approach to the question of whether limbic system dysfunction is related to subsequent carbamazepine response is based on the use of a pharmacological challenge with procaine. Procaine, like other local anesthetics, is thought to have some selectivity for activating limbic system structures (103). Although the mechanism of action of the local anesthetics is not known, we chose to employ procaine because of its record of safety when given intravenously to patients (Ken Livingston, personal communication), its short half-life, and the indirect evidence that it would provide some selectivity of excitation of limbic system structures. In the study, we hoped to answer two questions. First, was there an alteration in limbic system excitability or threshold among different diagnostic groups? Second, would differential responsivity to procaine predict subsequent re-

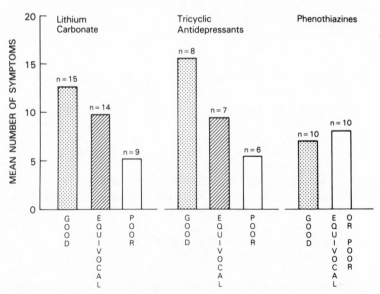

Figure 6. Relationship of Drug Response to Epileptic-Like Symptoms

sponse to carbamazepine? To date, we have studied 21 subjects with affective disorders, borderline personality disorders, or normal controls (142). In collaboration with R. Coppola we have established that procaine does, in fact, produce relatively selective activation of fast frequencies (28 to 40 Hz) in EEG over temporal lobes. This is the first confirmation in humans that the local anesthetics may, in fact, be exerting some selective activating effects in temporal lobe or limbic system structures. Kellner et al. (142) found that this agent induced more anxiety and dysphoria than euphoria and induced distortions of sensations in all sensory modalities. The degree of increase in fast activity over the temporal lobes was significantly ($p < .05$) correlated with the degree of depression (.48), anxiety (.57), and anger (.49). Moreover, the sensory and cognitive distortions appeared to occur in a dose-related fashion; in particular, complaints of ringing of the ears or tinnitus increased in frequency and intensity as a function of procaine dose. Some patients reported hallucinatory-like experiences, including two patients who reported smelling tuna fish. Two patients reported a recall of experientially vivid and immediate memories that were of such intensity that they appeared almost hallucinatory. Similar sensory and cognitive changes have been reported on direct stimulation of temporal lobe and limbic system structures in the studies of Penfield and Perot (143), Gloor et al. (23), and Halgren et al. (144). In addition to the EEG and psychosensory evidence that procaine was producing some activation of temporal lobe and limbic system structures, Kellner, Gold, and Kling (unpublished manuscript, 1985) observed a pattern of endocrine change consistent with the release of CRF. These investigators observed increases in plasma adrenocorticotropic hormone (ACTH), cortisol, and prolactin (but not growth hormone) following procaine administration. Thus this strategy holds promise as a probe of limbic system dysfunction and as a possible marker of subsequent carbamazepine response.

One further cautionary note is indicated in the interpretation of the procaine data, particularly if it turns out to be a predictor of carbamazepine response. The local anesthetic lidocaine also is a predictor of subsequent carbamazepine response in another syndrome that does not appear to involve limbic system dysfunction. Acute infusions of lidocaine are effective in treating myoclonic tinnitus and appear to be excellent predictors of subsequent long-term response to carbamazepine in this syndrome (145–148). Thus it would appear premature to conclude that response to a local anesthetic, even one purportedly causing appropriate excitation of limbic system structures, would necessarily imply limbic system pathology underlying a given disorder or that carbamazepine was effective by ameliorating such a dysfunction. Again, it would be possible for carbamazepine and the local anesthetics to share some common mechanism of action elsewhere in the brain that could lead to such a prediction.

ECT as an Anticonvulsant

The use of carbamazepine and related anticonvulsants in the treatment of primary and secondary affective illness allows a novel refocus on the mechanisms underlying the efficacy of ECT. How is it that both major motor seizures induced by electroconvulsive shock (ECS) and anticonvulsants are effective in the treatment of manic-depressive illness? One approach to this apparent paradox is based on our recent findings that ECS in the rat is, in fact, a potent anticonvulsant to limbic system seizures. In collaboration with Putnam and Contel (149) we observed ECS administered 6 hours prior to each amygdala kindling stimulation significantly, and essentially completely, inhibited the development of amygdala kindling compared to sham ECS controls. In contrast, active ECS given immediately after amygdala kindling was not effective in suppressing kindling development (149). In a separate series of studies, we also assessed the effects of ECS on completed kindled seizures. Animals were kindled to a point where they experienced a stage 4 seizure. Four groups of animals were then studied without further kindling over the next 7 days. ECS was given either on a once-daily basis for 7 days or given on a single occasion followed by a 6-day delay; each group had its sham ECS controls. Only in the group given ECS for 7 days was there a significant and long-lasting effect on kindling once amygdala stimulations were resumed. These data suggest that a series of chronic ECS in the rat exert a long-lasting anticonvulsant effect against amygdala kindling for up to 5 days following the termination of the series.

Taken together, these two studies, as well as those of Babington (116) and others in the literature (150), suggest that the major motor seizures achieved with ECT may in themselves be exerting potent anticonvulsant effects. Since we and others have observed that carbamazepine, while it is an effective acute anticonvulsant for amygdala-kindled seizures, does not prevent the development of amygdala kindling in the rat (149, 151) [as it does in the cat and monkey (152)], it would appear that ECS is an even more effective anticonvulsant than carbamazepine, at least on the development of amygdala kindling in the rat.

Thus it is possible that neurophysiologial or biochemical mechanisms achieved by ECS, which may be shared by anticonvulsants such as carbamazepine, can indirectly account for their common psychotropic effects in mania and depression. Although the mode of action of ECS is not known, our hypothesis gives a focused strategy for further research exploration on the possible mechanisms of action of ECS, with a focus on a clearcut endpoint of its anticonvulsant effects.

It is of particular interest to note that ECS has been reported to be effective in treating depression associated with parkinsonism and the motor oscillations in Parkinson's disease manifested by the on-off phenomenon (153). Therefore, seizures induced by ECT may have anticonvulsant properties, motor stabilizing effects, and positive psychotropic effects in primary and secondary affective illness.

CONCLUSIONS

Thus we have come full circle. Some types of seizures may predispose to psychopathology, while the major motor seizures of ECT may treat mood and motor dysregulation. As emphasized by Trimble (60), there may be both reciprocal and direct relationships between seizures and psychosis (and related forms of psychopathology). The anticonvulsants may provide a new leverage point in further dissecting these relationships and in indirectly spurring closer ties between the disciplines of neurology and psychiatry. New convulsive therapies and technologies should lead to better understanding of the anatomical, biochemical, and physiological underpinnings of dysregulated behavior. We have attempted to highlight some of the complexity and promise in the field of understanding the relationships between seizures and psychiatric disorders. Both seizures (of ECT) and anticonvulsants have now been borrowed from neurology in the service of better treatment of psychiatric patients. We look forward to further advances in the understanding and treatment of the disorders of brain function subsumed by both psychiatry and neurology.

REFERENCES

1. Jackson JH: On a case of loss of power of expression; inability to talk, to write, and to read correctly after convulsive attacks. Br Med J 11:326–330, 1866

2. Landolt A: Serial EEG investigations during psychotic episodes in epileptic patients and during schizophrenic attacks, in Lectures on Epilepsy. Edited by de Maas L. Amsterdam, Elsevier, 1958

3. von Meduna LJ: Die konvulsionstherapie der schizophrenie. Psychiatr Neurol Wochscher 37:317–319, 1935

4. Waxman SG, Geshwind N: The interictal behavior syndrome of epilepsy. Arch Gen Psychiatry 32:1580–1588, 1975

5. Bear DM, Fedio P: Quantitative analysis of interictal behavior in temporal lobe epilepsy. Arch Neurol 34:454–467, 1977

6. Bear DM. Temporal lobe epilepsy: a syndrome of sensory-limbic hyperconnection. Cortex 15:357–384, 1979

7. Bear DM, Leven K, Blumer D, et al: Interictal behavior in hospitalized temporal lobe epileptics: relationship to idopathic psychiatric syndromes. J Neurol Neurosurg Psychiatry 45:481–488, 1982

8. Stevens JR: Risk factors for psychopathology in individuals with epilepsy, in Advances in Biological Psychiatry: Temporal Lobe Epilepsy, Mania and Schizophrenia and the Limbic System. Edited by Koella WP, Trimble MR. Basel, S Karger, 1982

9. Mungus D: Interictal behavior abnormality in temporal lobe epilepsy: a specific syndrome or nonspecific psychopathology? Arch Gen Psychiatry 39:108–111, 1982

10. Hermann BP, Whitman S, Arnston P: Hypergraphia in epilepsy: is there a specificity to temporal lobe epilepsy? J Neurol Neurosurg Psychiatry 46:848–853, 1983

11. Hermann BP, Riel P: Interictal personality and behavioral traits in temporal lobe and generalized epilepsy. Cortex 17:125–128, 1981

12. Stark-Adamec C, Adamec R: Psychological methodology versus clinical impressions: different perspectives on psychopathology and seizures, in Patterns of Limbic System Dysfunction: Seizures, Psychosis, Discontrol. Edited by Doane BK. New York, Raven Press, 1984

13. Bellur S, Camacho A, Hermann B, et al: Autonomic responsiveness to affective visual stimulation in temporal lobe epilepsy. Biol Psychiatry 20:73–78, 1984

14. Post RM, Uhde TW: Treatment of mood disorders with antiepileptic medications: clinical and theoretical implications. Epilepsia 24:97–108, 1983

15. Post RM, Ballenger JC, Uhde TW, et al: Efficacy of carbamazepine in manic-depressive illness: implications for underlying mechanisms, in Neurobiology of Mood Disorders. Edited by Post RM, Ballenger JC. Baltimore, Williams & Wilkins, 1984, pp 777–816

16. Ballenger JC, Post RM: Carbamazepine (Tegretol) in manic-depressive illness: a new treatment. Am J Psychiatry 137:782–790, 1980

17. Post RM, Uhde TW, Roy-Byrne PP, et al: Antidepressant effects of carbamazepine. Am J Psychiatry (in press)

18. Post RM, Uhde TW, Ballenger JC, et al: Prophylactic efficacy of carbamazepine in manic-depressive illness. Am J Psychiatry 140:1602–1604, 1983

19. Okuma T, Inanaga K, Otsuki S, et al: A preliminary double-blind study of the efficacy of carbamazepine in prophylaxis of manic-depressive illness. Psychopharmacology 73:95–96, 1981

20. Gibbs F: Ictal and non-ictal psychiatric disorders in temporal lobe epilepsy. J Nerv Ment Dis 113:522–528, 1951

21. Slater E, Beard AW, Glithero E: The schizophrenia-like psychosis of epilepsy. Br J Psychiatry 109:95–150, 1963

22. Hermann BP, Dikmen S, Schwartz MS, et al: Interictal psychopathology in patients with ictal fear: a quantitative investigation. Neurology 32:7–11, 1982

23. Gloor P. Olivier A, Quesney LF, et al: The role of the limbic system in experiential phenomena of temporal lobe epilepsy. Ann Neurol 12:129–144, 1982

24. Flor-Henry P: Schizophrenic-like reactions and affective psychoses associated with temporal lobe epilepsy: etiological factors. Am J Psychiatry 126:400–404, 1969

25. Dongier S: Statistical study of clinical and electroencephalographic manifestations of 536 psychotic episodes occurring in 516 epileptics between clinical seizures. Epilepsia 1:117–142, 1960

26. Kristensen O, Sindrup EH: Psychomotor epilepsy and psychosis. Acta Neurol Scand 57:370–379, 1978

27. Perez MM, Trimble MR: Epileptic psychosis-diagnostic comparison with process schizophrenia. Br J Psychiatry 137:245–249, 1980

28. Glaser GH: The problem of psychosis in psychomotor epileptics. Epilepsia 5:271–278, 1964

29. Hill D: Psychiatric disorders of epilepsy. Medical Press 229:473–475, 1952

30. Pond DA: Psychiatric aspects of epilepsy. Journal of the Indian Medical Profession 3:1441–1451, 1957

31. Robertson MM, Trimble MR: Depressive illness in patients with epilepsy: a review. Epilepsia 24:109–116, 1983

31a. Spitzer RL, Endicott J, Robins E: Research Diagnostic Criteria (RDC) for a Selected Group of Functional Disorders. New York, New York State Psychiatric Institute, 1980

31b. American Psychiatric Association: Diagnostic and Statistical Manual of Mental Disorders. 3rd ed. Washington, DC, American Psychiatric Association, 1980

32. Betts TA: Depression, anxiety and epilepsy, in Epilepsy and Psychiatry. Edited by Reynolds EH, Trimble MR. Edinburgh, Churchill Livingstone, 1981, pp 60–71

33. Weil A: Ictal depression and anxiety in temporal lobe disorders. Am J Psychiatry 113:149–157, 1956

34. Williams D: The structure of emotions reflected in epileptic experiences. Brain 74:29–67, 1956

35. Robertson M: Depression and epilepsy. Proceedings of the 15th Epilepsy International Symposium, Washington, DC, 27 September 1983

36. Mignone RJ, Donnelly EF, Sadowsky D: Psychological and neurological comparisons of psychomotor and non-psychomotor epileptic patients. Epilepsia 11:345–359, 1970

37. Dominian J, Serafetinides EA, Dewhurst M: A follow-up study of late-onset epilepsy. II. Psychiatric and social findings. Br Med J 5328:421–435, 1963

38. Wolf P: Manic episodes in epilepsy, in Advances in Epileptology: the XIIIth Epilepsy International Symposium. Edited by Akimoto H, Kazamatsuri H, Seino M, et al. New York, Raven Press, 1982

39. Dalby MA: Antiepileptic and psychotropic effect of carbamazepine (Tegretol) in the treatment of psychomotor epilepsy. Epilepsia 12:325–334, 1971

40. Forrest DV: Bipolar illness after right hemispherectomy. Arch Gen Psychiatry 39:817–819, 1982

41. Flor-Henry P: Psychosis and temporal lobe epilepsy: a controlled investigation. Epilepsia 10:363–395, 1969

42. Harper M, Roth M: Temporal lobe epilepsy and the phobic anxiety-depersonalization syndrome. Compr Psychiatry 3:129–151, 1962

43. Jackson JH: On epilepsy and epileptiform convulsions, in Selected Writings of John Hughlings Jackson. Edited by Taylor J, Holmes G, Walshe FMR. London, Hodder & Stoughton Ltd, 1931

44. Daly D: Ictal affect. Am J Psychiatry 115:97–108, 1958

45. Henriksen GF: Status epilepticus partialis with fear as clinical expression. Epilepsia 14:39–46, 1973

46. McLachlan RS, Blume WT: Isolated fear in complex partial status epilepticus. Ann Neurol 8:639–641, 1980

47. Mullan S, Penfield W: Illusions of comparative interpretation and emotion. Arch Neurol Psychiatry 81:269–284, 1959

48. Heath RG, Monroe RR, Mickle W: Stimulation of the amygdaloid nucleus in a schizophrenic patient. Am J Psychiatry 111:862–863, 1955

49. Mulder DW, Daly D: Psychiatric symptoms associated with lesions of the temporal lobe. JAMA 150:173–176, 1952

50. Currie S, Heathfield KWG, Henson RA, et al: Clinical course and prognosis of temporal lobe epilepsy. Brain 94:173–190, 1971

51. Penfield W: The role of the temporal cortex in certain psychical phenomena: 29th Maudsley Lecture. Journal of Mental Science 101:451–465, 1955

52. Brodsky L, Zuniga JS, Casenas ER, et al: Refractory anxiety: a masked epileptiform disorder? Psychiatr J Univ Ottawa 8:42–45, 1983

53. Hilton SM, Zbrozyna AW: Amygdaloid region for defense reactions and its efferent pathway to the brain stem. J Physiol (London) 165:160–173, 1963

54. Fonberg E: Effect of partial destruction of the amygdaloid complex on the emotional defensive behaviour of dogs. Bulletin Academie Polonaise des Sciences Biologiques 13:429–432, 1965

55. Egger MD, Flynn JP: Further studies on the effects of amygdaloid stimulation and ablation in hypothalamically elicited attack behavior in cats, in Structure and Function of the Limbic System (Progress in Brain Research, Vol 27). Edited by Adey WR, Tokizane T. Amsterdam, Elsevier, 1967, pp 165–182

56. Belluzzi JD, Grossman SP: Avoidance learning: long lasting deficits after temporal lobe seizure. Science 166:1435–1437, 1969

57. Pincus JH: Can violence be a manifestation of epilepsy. Neurology 30:304–307, 1980

58. Sherwin I: The effect of the location of an epileptogenic lesion on the occurrence of psychosis in epilepsy, in Advances in Biological Psychiatry, Vol 8: Temporal Lobe Epilepsy, Mania, and Schizophrenia and the Limbic System. Edited by Koella WP, Trimble MR. Basel, S Karger, 1982, pp 81–97

59. Lindsay J, Ounsted C, Richards P: Long-term outcome in children with temporal lobe seizures. III Psychiatric aspects in childhood and adult life. Dev Med Child Neurol 21:630–636, 1979

60. Trimble MR: Interictal psychoses of epilepsy. Acta Psychiatr Scand 69(Suppl 313):9–20, 1984

61. Bruens JH: Psychoses in epilepsy: historic concepts and new developments, in Advances in Epileptology: XIth Epilepsy Internat Symposium. Edited by Canger R, Angeleri F, Penry JK. New York, Raven Press, 1980, pp 161–166

62. Macrae D: Isolated fear: a temporal lobe aura. Neurology 4:497–505, 1954

63. Small JG, Milstein V, Klapper MH, et al: ECT in the treatment of manic disorders. Ann NY Acad Sci (in press)

64. Perini G, Mendius R: Depression and anxiety in complex partial seizures. J Nerv Ment Dis 172:287–290, 1984

65. Trimble MR, Perez MM: The phenomenology of the chronic psychoses of epilepsy, in Seizures, Psychosis, Mania and the Hippo Link. Edited by Koella W, Trimble MR. Basel, S Karger, 1982, pp 98–105

66. McIntyre M, Pritchard PB, Lombroso CT: Left and right temporal lobe epileptics: a controlled investigation of some psychological differences. Epilepsia 17:377–386, 1976

67. Serafetinides EA: Aggressiveness in temporal lobe epileptics and its relation to cerebral dysfunction and environmental factors. Epilepsia 6:33–42, 1965

68. Sackeim HA, Greenberg MS, Weiman AL, et al: Hemispheric asymmetry in the expression of positive and negative emotions: neurological evidence. Arch Neurol 39:210–218, 1982

69. Kolb B, Taylor L: Affective behavior in patients with localized cortical excisions: role of lesion site and side. Science 214:89–90, 1981

70. Engel J Jr, Kuhl DE, Phelps ME: Patterns of human local cerebral glucose metabolism during epileptic seizures. Science 218:64–66, 1982

71. Gale K, Engel J, Ferrendelli J, et al: Brain circuitry involved in convulsant and anticonvulsant processes. Proceedings of the 18th Annual Winter Conference on Brain Research, Vail, Colorado, 26 January–2 February 1985

72. Sherwin I: Psychosis associated with epilepsy: significance of the laterality of the epileptogenic lesion. J Neurol Neurosurg Psychiatry 44:83–85, 1981

73. Stevens JR: Biological background of psychosis in epilepsy, in Advances in Epileptology: XIth Epilepsy Internat Symposium. Edited by Canger R, Angeleri F, Penry JK. New York, Raven Press, 1980, pp 167–172

74. Jensen I, Larsen JK: Mental aspects of temporal lobe epilepsy: follow-up of 74 patients after resection of a temporal lobe. J Neurol Neurosurg Psychiatry 42:256–265, 1979

75. Taylor DC: Factors influencing the occurrence of schizophrenia-like psychosis in patients with temporal lobe epilepsy. Psychol Med 5:249–254, 1979

76. Wolf P: Psychic disorders in epilepsy, in Advances in Epileptology: XIth Epilepsy Internat Symposium. Edited by Canger R, Angeleri F, Penry JK. New York, Raven Press, 1980, pp 159–160

77. Ramani V, Gumnit RJ: Intensive monitoring of epileptic patients with a history of episodic aggression. Arch Neurol 38:570–571, 1981

78. Trimble MR: The relationship between epilepsy and schizophrenia: a biochemical hypothesis. Biol Psychiatry 12:299–304, 1977

79. Alving J: Classification of the epilepsies: an investigation of 1,508 consecutive adult patients. Acta Neurol Scand 58:205–212, 1978

80. Valenstein E: the interpretation of behavior evoked by brain stimulation reward, in Brain-Stimulation Reward. Edited by Wauquier A, Rolls E. New York, Elsevier, 1976, pp 557–575

81. Kopa J, Szabo I, Grastyan E: A dual behavioral effect from stimulating the same thalamic point with identical stimulus parameter in different conditional reflex situations, in Biological Foundations of Emotion. Edited by Gellhorn E. Chicago, Scott, Foresman & Co., 1968, pp 107–127

82. Belenkov NY, Shalkovskaya LN: Role of dominant motivation in manifestation of the effects of electrical stimulation of the hypothalamus and limbic region. Neurosci Behav Physiol 10:112–117, 1980

83. Penfield W, Rasmussen T: The Cerebral Cortex of Man. New York, Macmillan, 1950, p 164

84. Goddard GV, McIntyre DC, Leech CK: A permanent change in brain function resulting from daily electrical stimulation. Exp Neurol 25:295–330, 1969

85. Pinel JPJ: Kindling-induced experimental epilepsy in rats: cortical stimulation. Exp Neurol 72:559–569, 1981

86. Post RM, Kopanda RT, Lee A: Progressive behavioral changes during chronic lidocaine administration: relationship to kindling. Life Sci 17:943–950, 1975

87. Adamec R: Behavioral and epileptic determinants of predatory attack behavior in the cat. Can J Neurol Sci 2:457–466, 1975

88. Post RM, Kopanda RT: Cocaine, kindling, and psychosis. Am J Psychiatry 133:627–634, 1976

89. Post RM: Clinical implications of a cocaine-kindling model of psychosis, in Clinical Neuropharmacology, Vol 11. Edited by Klawans HL. New York, Raven Press, 1977, pp 25–42

90. Woodruff ML: Subconvulsive epileptiform discharge and behavioral impairment. Behavioral Biology 11:431–458, 1974

91. Bear D, Schenk L, Benson H: Increased autonomic responses to neutral and emotional stimuli in patients with temporal lobe epilepsy. Am J Psychiatry 138:843–845, 1981

92. Slater E, Moran PAP: The schizophrenia-like psychoses of epilepsy: relation between ages of onset. Br J Psychiatry 115:599–600, 1969

93. Pritchard PB, Lombrose CT, McIntyre M: Psychological complications of temporal lobe epilepsy. Neurology 30:227–232, 1980

94. Ehlers CL, Koob GF, Henriksen SJ, et al: Changes in locomotor activity in rats 'kindled' in the amygdala and nucleus accumbens septi [abstract no. 137.2]. Society for Neuroscience Abstracts 6:399, 1980

95. Pinel JPJ, Treit D, Royner LI: Temporal lobe aggression in rats. Science 197:1088–1089, 1977

96. Bawden HN, Racine RJ: Effects of bilateral kindling or bilateral subthreshold stimulation of the amygdala or septum on muricide, ranacide, intraspecific aggression and passive avoidance in the rat. Physiol Behav 22:115–123, 1979

97. Weiss SRB, Post RM, Gold PW, et al: CRF-induced seizures and behavior: interaction with amygdala kindling. Brain Res (in press)

98. Gold PW, Chrousos GP, Kellner CK, et al: Psychiatric implications of basic and clinical studies with corticotropin-releasing factor. Am J Psychiatry 141:619–627, 1984

99. Post RM, Kennedy C, Shinohara M, et al: Metabolic and behavioral consequences of lidocaine-kindled seizures. Brain Res 324:295–303, 1984

100. Mellanby J: Kindling, behaviour and anticonvulsant drugs. Clin Neuropharmacol 7:258, 1984

101. Post RM, Ballenger JC: Kindling models for the progressive development of behavioral psychopathology: sensitization to electrical, pharmacological, and psychological stimuli, in Handbook of Biological Psychiatry, Part IV. Edited by van Praag HM, Lader MH, Rafaelsen OJ, Sachar EJ. New York, Marcel-Dekker, 1981, pp 609–651

102. Post RM, Lockfeld A, Squillace KM, et al: Drug-environment interaction: context dependency of cocaine-induced behavioral sensitization. Life Sci 28:755–760, 1981

103. Post RM, Weiss SRB, Pert A, et al: Chronic cocaine administration: sensitization and kindling effects. American College of Neuropsychopharmacology (in press)

104. Washton AM, Gold MS: Chronic cocaine abuse: evidence for adverse effects on health and functioning. Psychiatric Annals 14:733–743, 1984

105. Deneau GA, Yanagita T, Seevers MH: Self administration of psychoactive substances by the monkey. Psychopharmacologia 16:30–48, 1969

106. Post RM: Clinical aspects of cocaine: assessment of acute and chronic effects in animals and man, in Cocaine: Chemical, Biological, Clinical, Social, and Treatment Aspects. Edited by Mule SJ. Cleveland, CRC Press, 1976, pp 203–215

107. Washton AM, Tatarsky A: Adverse effects of cocaine abuse, in Problems of Drug Dependence, 1983. NIDA Research Monograph 49. Edited by Harris LS. Washington, DC, US Government Printing Office, 1984, pp 247–254

108. Ballenger JC, Post RM: Kindling as a model for the alcohol withdrawal syndromes. Br J Psychiatry 133:1–14, 1978

109. Ballenger JC, Post RM: Carbamazepine in alcohol withdrawal syndromes and schizophrenic psychoses. Psychopharmacol Bull 20:572–584, 1984

110. Dackis CA, Stuckey RF: Psychopharmacologic treatment of the alcoholic. Fair Oaks Hospital Psychiatry Letter 2(7) 1984

111. Bolwig TG: Kindling as a model for alcohol withdrawal syndromes in the rat. Presented at the NIMH Biological Psychiatry Branch Meeting, Bethesda, Maryland, 24 January

112. Post R, Ballenger J, Putnam F, et al: Carbamazepine in alcohol withdrawal syndromes: relationship to the kindling model. J Clin Psychopharmacol 3:204–205, 1983

113. Dalby MA: Behavioral effects of carbamazepine, in Complex Partial Seizures and Their Treatment: Advances in Neurology, Vol 11. Edited by Penry JK, Daly DD. New York, Raven Press, 1975, pp 331–344

114. Hernandez-Peon R: Anticonvulsive action of G 32883, in Neuropsychopharmacology, Vol 3. Edited by Bradley PB, Flugel F, Hoch PH. Amsterdam, Elsevier, 1964, pp 303–311

115. Koella WP, Levin P, Baltzer V: The pharmacology of carbamazepine and some other anti-epileptic drugs, in Epileptic Seizures, Behavior, Pain. Edited by Birkmayer W. Bern, Hans Huber, 1976, pp 32–50

116. Babington RG: The pharmacology of kindling, in Animal Models of Psychiatry and Neurology. Edited by Hanin I, Usdin E. New York, Pergamon Press, 1977, pp 141–149

117. Albright PS, Burnham WM: Development of a new pharmacological seizure model: effects of anticonvulsants on cortical- and amygdala-kindled seizures in the rat. Epilepsia 21:681–689, 1980

118. Penry JK, Daly DD: Complex Partial Seizures and Their Treatment: Advances in Neurology, Vol 11. New York, Raven Press, 1975

119. Porter RJ, Penry JK: Efficacy and choice of antiepileptic drugs, in Advances in Epileptology, 1977: Psychology, Pharmacotherapy, and New Diagnostic Approaches. Edited by Meinardi H, Rowan AJ. Amsterdam, Swets & Zeitlinger, 1978, pp 220–230

120. Takezaki H, Hanaoka M: The use of carbamazepine (Tegretol) in the control of manic-depressive psychosis and other manic, depressive states. Clinical Psychiatry 13:173–183, 1971

121. Okuma T, Kishimoto A, Inoue K, et al: Anti-manic and prophylactic effects of carbamazepine on manic-depressive psychosis. Folia Psychiatr Neurol Jpn 27:283–297, 1973

122. Post RM, Uhde TW: The use of carbamazepine in mania, in Drugs in Psychiatry, Vol 4: Antimanics, Anticonvulsants, and Other Drugs in Psychiatry. Edited by Burrows GD, Norman TR, Davies D. Amsterdam, Elsevier (in press)

123. Post RM, Uhde TW, Ballenger JC: Efficacy of carbamazepine in affective disorders: implications for underlying physiological and biochemical substrates, in Anticonvulsants in Affective Disorders. Edited by Emrich HM, Okuma T, Muller AA. Amsterdam, Elsevier, 1984, pp 93–115

124. Ramsey RE, Wilder BJ, Berger JR, et al: A double-blind study comparing carbamazepine with phenytoin as initial seizure therapy in adults. Neurology 33:904–910, 1983

125. Porter RJ, Theodore WH: Nonsedative regimens in the treatment of epilepsy. Arch Intern Med 143:945–947, 1983

126. Lambert PA: Acute and prophylactic therapies of patients with affective disorders using valpromide (dipropylacetamide), in Anticonvulsants in Affective Disorders. Edited by Emrich HM, Okuma T, Muller AA. Amsterdam, Elsevier, 1984, pp 33–44

127. Emrich HM, von Zerssen D, Kissling W, et al: Effect of sodium valproate in mania. The GABA-hypothesis of affective disorders. Archiv fuer Psychiatrie und Nervenkrankenheiten 229:1–16, 1980

128. Emrich HM, Stoll K-D, Muller AA: Guidelines for the use of carbamazepine and of valproate in the prophylaxis of affective disorders, in Anticonvulsants in Affective Disorders. Edited by Emrich HM, Okuma T, Muller AA. Amsterdam, Elsevier, 1984, pp 211–214

129. Puzynski S, Klosiewicz L: Valproic acid as a prophylactic agent in affective and schizoaffective disorders, in Anticonvulsants in Affective Disorders. Edited by Emrich HM, Okuma T, Muller AA. Amsterdam, Elsevier, 1984, pp 68–75

130. Vencovsky E, Soucek K, Kabes J: Prophylactic effect of dipropylacetamide in patients with bipolar affective disorder: short communication, in Anticonvulsants in Affective Disorders. Edited by Emrich HM, Okuma T, Muller AA. Amsterdam, Elsevier, 1984, pp 66–67

131. Brennan MJW, Sandyk R, Barsook D: Use of sodium-valproate in the management of affective disorders: basic and clinical aspects, in Anticonvulsants in Affective Disorders. Edited by Emrich HM, Okuma T, Muller AA. Amsterdam, Elsevier, 1984, pp 56–65

132. Kalinowsky LB, Putnam TJ: Attempts at treatment of schizophrenia and other non-epileptic psychoses with dilantin. Archives of Neurology and Psychiatry 49:414–420, 1943

133. Kubanek JL, Rowell RC: The use of dilantin on the treatment of psychotic patients unresponsive to other treatment. Diseases of the Nervous System 7:47–50, 1946

134. Freyhan FA: Effectiveness of diphenylhydantoin in management of nonepileptic psychomotor excitement states. Archives of Neurology and Psychiatry 53:370–374, 1945

135. Dreyfus J: A Remarkable Medicine Has Been Overlooked. New York, Simon and Schuster, 1981

136. Phelps ME: The biochemical basis of cerebral function and its investigation in humans with positron CT. Proceedings of the American Psychiatric Association 137th Annual Meeting, Los Angeles, 5–11 May 1984, p 11

137. Silberman EK, Post RM, Nurnberger J, et al: Epileptic-like symptoms in affective illness. Abstracts of the American Psychiatric Association, 4 May 1983

138. Silberman E, Post RM, Nurnberger J, et al: Transient sensory, cognitive, and affective phenomena in affective illness: a comparison with complex partial epilepsy. Br J Psychiatry 146:881–889, 1985

139. Mueller PS, Allen NG: Diagnosis and treatment of severe light-sensitive seasonal energy syndrome (SES) and its relationship to melatonin anabolism. Fair Oaks Hospital Psychiatry Letter 11(9) 1984

140. Uhde TW, Boulenger J-P, Roy-Byrne PP, et al: Longitudinal course of panic disorder: clinical and biological considerations. Prog Neuropsychopharmacol Biol Psychiatry 9:39–51, 1985

141. Chapman J: the early symptoms of schizophrenia. Br J Psychiatry 112:225–251, 1966

142. Kellner CH, Kling M, Post RM, et al: Intravenous procaine as a probe of limbic activity. New Research Abstracts, American Psychiatric Association, Annual Meeting, Dallas, 18–24 May 1985

143. Penfield W, Perot P: The brain's record of auditory and visual experience: a final summary and discussion. Brain 86:595–696, 1963

144. Halgren E, Walter RD, Cherlow DG, et al: Mental phenomena evoked by electrical stimulation of the human hippocampal formation and amygdala. Brain 101:83–117, 1978

145. Shea JJ, Harell M: Management of tinnitus aurium with lidocaine and carbamazepine. Laryngoscope 88:1477, 1978

146. Rahko T, Hakkinen V: Carbamazepine in the treatment of objective myoclonus tinnitus. J Laryngol Otol 93:123–127, 1979

147. Melding PS, Goodey RJ: The treatment of tinnitus with oral anticonvulsants. J Laryngol Otol 93:111–122, 1979

148. Hess JC, Viada J, May A: Evaluacion de la prueba de la lidocaina y del tratamiento con carbamazepine in pacientes con tinnitus. Rev Laryngol Otol Rhinol (Bord) 40:5–10, 1980

149. Post RM, Putnam F, Contel NR, et al: Electroconvulsive seizures inhibit amygdala kindling: implications for mechanisms of action in affective illness. Epilepsia 25:234–239, 1984

150. Post RM, Putnam F, Uhde TW, et al: ECT as an anticonvulsant: implications for its mechanism of action in affective illness. Ann NY Acad Sci (in press)

151. Balster V, Klebs K, Schmutz M: Effects of oxcarbazepine, a compound related to carbamazepine, and of GP47 779, its main metabolite in man, on the evolution of amygdaloid-kindled seizures in the rat. Presented at Epilepsy International Congress, Kyoto, Japan, 17–21 September 1981

152. Wada JA, Sato M, Wake A, et al: Prophylactic effects of phenytoin, phenobarbital, and carbamazepine examined in kindled cat preparations. Arch Neurol 33:426–434, 1976

153. Coffey CE, Ross DR, Ferren BS, et al: Treatment of the "on-off" phenomenon in parkinsonism and lithium carbonate. Ann Neurol 12:375–379, 1982

154. Matthews CG, Klove H: MMPI performances in major motor, psychomotor and mixed seizure classifications of known and unknown etiology. Epilepsia 9:43–53, 1968

155. Glass DH, Mattson RH: Psychopathology and emotional precipitation of seizures in temporal lobe epileptics. Proceedings of the 81st Annual Meeting of the American Psychological Association, Vol 8, 1973, p 425

156. Standage KF, Fenton GW: Psychiatric symptom profiles of patients with epilepsy: a controlled investigation. Psychol Med 5:152–160, 1975

157. Rodin EA, Katz M, Lennox K: Differences between patients with temporal lobe seizures and those with other forms of epileptic attacks. Epilepsia 17:313–320, 1976

158. Taylor DC: Mental state and temporal lobe epilepsy: a correlative account of 100 patients treated surgically. Epilepsia 13:727–765, 1972

159. Shukla GD, Srivastava ON, Katiyar BC, et al: Psychiatric manifestations in temporal lobe epilepsy: a controlled study. Br J Psychiatry 135:411–417, 1979

160. Small JG, Small IF, Hayden MP: Further psychiatric investigations of patients with temporal and nontemporal lobe epilepsy. Am J Psychiatry 123:303–310, 1966

161. Parnas J, Korsgaard S, Krautwald O, et al: Chronic psychosis in epilepsy. Acta Psychiatr Scand 66:282–293, 1982

162. Gregoriadis A, Fragos E, Kapsalakis Z, et al: A correlation between mental disorders and EEG and AEG findings in temporal lobe epilepsy. Proceedings of the 5th World Congress of Psychiatry, Mexico, 1971

163. Hara T, Hoshi A, Takase M, et al: Factors related to psychiatric episodes in epileptics. Folia Psychiatr Neurol Jpn 34:329–330, 1980

164. Toone BK, Dawson J, Driver MV: Psychoses of epilepsy: a radiological evaluation. Br J Psychiatry 140:244–248, 1982

165. Ounsted C, Lindsay J: The long-term outcome of temporal lobe epilepsy in childhood, in Epilepsy and Psychiatry. Edited by Reynolds EH, Trimble MR. Edinburgh, Churchill Livingstone, 1981, pp 185–215

166. Stevens JR: Psychomotor epilepsy and schizophrenia: a common anatomy?, in Epilepsy: Its Phenomena in Man. Edited by Brazier MAB. New York, Academic Press, 1973, pp 190–214

167. Ashford J, Wesson S, Schulz C, et al: Violent automatism in a partial complex seizure. Arch Neurol 37:120–122, 1980

168. Rodin EA: Psychomotor epilepsy and aggressive behavior. Arch Gen Psychiatry 28:210–213, 1973

169. Delgado-Escueta A, Mattson RH, King L, et al: The nature of aggression during epileptic seizures. N Engl J Med 305:711–716, 1981

170. Cirignotta F, Todesco CV, Lugaresi E: Temporal lobe epilepsy with ecstatic seizures (so-called Dostoevsky Epilepsy). Epilepsia 21:705–710, 1980

171. Mesulam MM: Dissociative states with abnormal temporal lobe EEG (multiple personality and the illusion of possession). Arch Neurol 38:176–181, 1981

172. Flor-Henry P: Lateralized temporal-limbic dysfunction and psychopathology. Ann NY Acad Sci 280:777–797, 1976

173. Mandell AJ: Toward a psychobiology of transcendence: God in the brain, in The Psychobiology of Consciousness. Edited by Davidson RJ, Davidson JM. New York, Plenum Press, 1980, pp 379–464

174. Heath RG: Pleasure response of human subjects to direct stimulation of the brain: physiologic and psychodynamic considerations, in The Role of Pleasure in Behavior. Edited by Heath RG. New York, Hoeber, 1964, pp 219–243

175. Schenk L, Bear D: Multiple personality disorder and related dissociative phenomena in patients with temporal lobe epilepsy. Am J Psychiatry 138:1311–1315, 1981

176. Tharp BR: Transient global amnesia: manifestation of medial temporal lobe epilepsy (letter). Clin Electroencephalogr 10:54–56, 1979

177. Penfield W: The Mystery of the Mind. A Critical Study of Consciousness and the Human Brain. Princeton, Princeton University Press, 1975

178. Jackson JH, Stewart P: Epileptic attacks with a warning of a crude sensation of smell and with the intellectual aura (dreamy state) in a patient who had symptoms pointing to gross organic disease of the right temporo-sphenoidal lobe. Brain 22:534–549, 1899

179. Wada JA, Sato M: Generalized convulsive seizures induced by daily electrical stimulation of the amygdala in cats. Neurology 24:565–574, 1974

180. Wada JA, Sato M, Corcoran ME: Persistent seizure susceptibility and recurrent spontaneous seizures in kindled cats. Epilepsia 15:465–478, 1974

181. Racine RJ: Kindling: the first decade. Neurosurgery 3:234–252, 1978

182. Pinel JPJ, Rovner LI: Electrode placement and kindling-induced experimental epilepsy. Exp Neurol 58:335–346, 1978

183. Pinel JPJ, Rovner LI: Experimental epileptogenesis: kindling-induced epilepsy in rats. Exp Neurol 58:190–202, 1978

184. Yde A, Lohse E, Faurbye A: On the relation between schizophrenia, epilepsy, and induced convulsions. Acta Psychiatr Neurol Scand 16:325–388, 1941

185. Gastaut H: Etude electroclinique des episodes psychotiques survenant en dehors des crises cliniques chez les epileptiques. Rev Neurol (Paris) 95:588–594, 1956

186. Serafetinides EA, Falconer MA: The effects of temporal lobectomy in epileptic patients with psychosis. Journal of Mental Science 108:584–593, 1962

187. Jus A: Troubles mentaux a symptomatologie schizophrenique chez les epileptiques. Evolution Psychiatrique 31:313–319, 1966

188. Bruens JH: Psychoses in epilepsy. Psychiatria Neurologia Neurochirurgia 74:175–192, 1971

189. Standage KF: Schizophreniform psychosis among epileptics in a mental hospital. Br J Psychiatry 123:321–232, 1973

190. Trixler M, Nador G: Schizophrenia-like psychoses in temporal lobe epilepsy. Electroencephalogr Clin Neurophysiol 41:213–214, 1976

191. Peters JG: Dopamine, noradrenaline and serotonin spinal fluid metabolites in temporal lobe epileptic patients with schizophrenic symptomatology. European Neurology 18:15–18, 1979

192. Sugano K, Miyasaka M: Epileptic psychosis and the occurring conditions. Folia Psychiatr Neurol Jpn 34:340–342, 1980

193. Ramani V, Gumnit RJ: Intensive monitoring of interictal psychosis in epilepsy. Ann Neurol 11:613–622, 1982

194. Post RM, Squillace KM, Pert A, et al: The effect of amygdala kindling on spontaneous and cocaine-induced motor activity and lidocaine seizures. Psychopharmacology 72:189–196, 1981

195. Weingartner H, White N: Exploration evoked by electrical stimulation of the amygdala of rats. Physiological Psychology 6:229–235, 1978

196. Innes EB, Locatell-Innes EM, Cornell JM: Amygdaloid kindled convulsions and modification of weight gains in hooded rats. Physiol Behav 18:187–192, 1977

197. McIntyre DC: Kindling and memory: the adrenal system and the bisected brain, in Limbic Mechanisms: The Continuing Evolution of the Limbic Concept. Edited by Livingston KE, Hornykiewicz O. New York, Plenum Press, 1978, pp 495–506

198. Yoshi N, Yamaguchi Y: Conditioning of seizure discharges with electrical stimulation of the limbic structures in cat. Folia Psychiatr Neurol Jpn 17:276–286, 1963

199. Gunne LM, Reis DJ: Changes in brain catecholamines associated with electrical stimulation of amygdaloid nucleus. Life Sci 2:804–809, 1963

200. Deflorida FA, Delgado JMR: Lasting behavioral and EEG changes in cats induced by prolonged stimulation of amygdala. Am J Psysiol 193:223–229, 1958

201. Boast CA, McIntyre DC: Bilateral kindled amygdala foci and inhibitory avoidance behavior in rats: a functional lesion effect. Physiol Behav 18:25–28, 1977

202. McIntyre DC, Molino A: Amygdala lesions and CER learning: long term effect of kindling. Physiol Behav 8:1055–1058, 1972

203. Heath RG, Monroe RR, Mickle W: Stimulation of the amygdaloid nucleus in a schizophrenic patient. Am J Psychiatry 111:862–863, 1955

204. Ervin FR, Delgado J, Mark VH, et al: Rage: a paraepileptic phenomenon? Epilepsia 10:417, 1969

205. Stevens JR, Mark VH, Erwin F, et al: Deep temporal stimulation in man. Arch Neurol 21:157–167, 1969

206. Goddard GV, Morrell F: Chronic progressive epileptogenesis induced by focal electrical stimulation of brain. Neurology 21:393, 1971

207. Stokes KA, McIntyre DC: Lateralized asymmetrical state-dependent learning produced by kindled convulsions from the rat hippocampus. Physiol Behav 26:163–169, 1981

208. Stevens JR, Livermore A Jr: Kindling of the mesolimbic dopamine system: animal model of psychosis. Neurology 28:36–46, 1978

209. Delgado JMR, Anand BK: Increase of food intake induced by electrical stimulation of the lateral hypothalamus. Am J Physiol 172:162–168, 1953

210. Valenstein ES, Cox VC, Kakolewski JW: Re-examination of the role of the hypothalamus in motivation. Psychol Rev 77:16, 1970

211. Wise RA: Hypothalamic motivational systems: fixed or plastic neural circuits. Science 162:377–379, 1968

Chapter 4

Primary Hypothyroidism and Its Relationship to Affective Disorders

Frederick C. Goggans, M.D.
R. Michael Allen, M.D.
Mark S. Gold, M.D.

Chapter 4

Primary Hypothyroidism and Its Relationship to Affective Disorders

The term "depression" may indicate either a symptom or a full behavioral syndrome. In either sense depression may also be a primary condition or may be a secondary manifestation of some other medical or psychiatric disorder. Recent evidence that will be discussed in this chapter suggests that early hypothyroidism may be the most common medical disorder that may mimic primary major depression. During the past decade our clinical and basic understanding of primary hyperthyroidism has changed our conceptualization of this disorder from an all-or-none construct to one in which the illness is seen as being present in at least three grades from subclinical to overt (1, 2). Routine thyroid tests may not identify the majority of patients early in the course of emerging thyroid dysfunction. Therefore psychiatrists should be aware of the physiology of the brain-thyroid axis as well as those newer tests that are able to aid the physician detect and grade primary thyroid dysfunction.

THE HYPOTHALAMIC-PITUITARY-THYROID AXIS

The thyroid gland is but one link in the neuroendocrine system known as the hypothalamic-pituitary-thyroid (HPT) axis (Figure 1). Within this axis circulating thyroid hormones are closely regulated by both central nervous system input and peripheral feedback control (3). The hypothalamus secretes a tripeptide hormone called thyrotropin-releasing hormone (TRH) into the portal hypophyseal circulation, which then transports TRH to the pituitary gland (4). The release of TRH is influenced by input from the limbic system, other areas in the central nervous system, and probably also from circulating levels of TRH itself and thyroid hormones in the brain and the pituitary (5). TRH acts at specific receptors on the anterior pituitary gland to cause the release of thyroid-stimulating hormone (TSH) into the circulation. TSH in turn acts on the thyroid gland itself to promote the release of thyroid hormones into the peripheral circulation. Serum thyroid hormone levels serve as a long feedback mechanism to modulate the release of TSH by the pituitary gland probably through an altering of the sensitivity of TRH receptors on the pi-

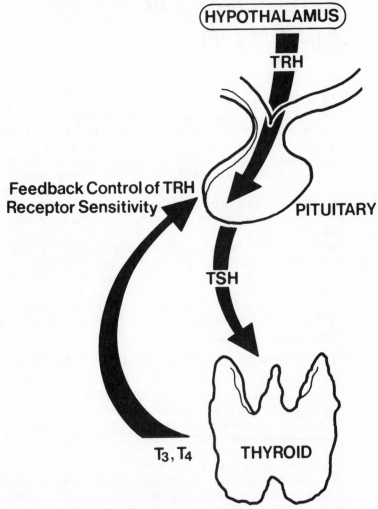

Figure 1. Schematic Representation of the Hypothalmic-Pituitary-Thyroid (HPT) Axis

tuitary. For example, as the levels of thyroid hormones decline from their usual equilibrium in a given individual with early thyroid failure, TSH receptors become suprasensitive to TRH stimulation and a proportionately higher amount of TSH is released. These changes are homeostatic attempts to compensate and to promote increased release of thyroid hormones from the thyroid gland. Levels of the thyroid hormones are maintained within the wide range of laboratory normals as long as the gland itself has enough synthetic reserve, but they could be lower compared to that individual's prior equilibrium point. This reduction in a particular individual's normal levels of thyroid hormones results in increased TRH receptor sensitivity and more TSH released per available molecule of TRH. As will be discussed below, changes of this kind within the HPT axis that result in "chemical" or "subclinical" hypothyroidism can be detected by measurement of serum TSH levels and by the TRH stimulation test. Whereas the classic endocrinologist who is concerned with myxedema and related syndromes of gross thyroid dysfunction may be less concerned with chemical or subclinical hypothyroidism, the psychiatrist or neurobehaviorally oriented clinician may see these states as relevant to the understanding and treatment of certain mental syndromes, especially those presenting with depression or mental lethargy.

THYROID HORMONES AND THEIR LABORATORY EVALUATION

Thyroxine, Triiodothyronine, and T3 Resin Uptake

There are two active forms of circulating thyroid hormone: L-thyroxine (T4) and triiodothyronine (T3). The thyroid gland secretes primarily but not exclusively T4. At least one-third of this T4 is converted by peripheral tissues to T3, which is now felt to be responsible for most of the biological effectiveness of the thyroid gland. Although T4 is secreted at nearly 10 times the rate of T3, T3 is 3 to 4 times more potent. Both of these hormones are bound to serum proteins, such as thyroid-binding globulin and thyroid-binding prealbumin. Therefore only a small amount of the total pool of circulating hormones is actually free in the serum and available to bind receptor sites. Synthesis of these hormones within the thyroid gland requires the presence of dietary iodide and the essential amino acid tyrosine. Although at one time a dietary deficiency of iodide was responsible for many cases of hypothyroidism in the United States, the addition of iodide to salt, bread, and other packaged foods has virtually eliminated this as an etiology of hypothyroidism today. By far the most common cause of hypothyroidism today is autoimmune thyroiditis, once termed Hashimoto's disease.

Circulating thyroid hormones used to be measured by protein-bound iodine or column chromatography. These methods are only of historical interest today. Currently the most commonly used assays for T4 are radioimmunoassay and competitive protein binding. Because both of these techniques measure total T4, they are influenced by changes in protein bindings sites. The T4 level obtained by these assays is therefore increased by conditions such as pregnancy, hepatitis, and the effects of medications such as estrogens; it is decreased by such conditions as nephrotic syndrome, major physical illness, and the presence of medications such as phenytoin (6). To help correct for these changes in binding capacity, the T3 resin uptake (T3RU) determination is performed. Essentially this is a measurement of the total thyroid hormone-binding sites available. In this test a standard amount of the patient's serum is mixed with radioactively labeled T3 and with a resin that absorbs thyroid hormones. The labeled T3, which is not absorbed by binding sites in the patient's serum, is absorbed by the added resin, which is then measured. If the patient has an excess of thyroid hormone (i.e., is hyperthyroid) or a decrease in binding sites, most of the binding sites are filled and there is a surplus of labeled T3 absorbed by the resin. The converse is true in hypothyroidism or when binding sites are increased. Therefore an increase in the T3RU indicates a decrease in available binding sites and a decrease in the T3RU indicates an increase in available binding sites. If one computes the product of total T4 and the T3RU, one obtains the free thyroxine index (FTI), which gives a more accurate value for the level of free circulating hormone. This calculated value correlates well with free T4 as measured by dialysis.

TSH

The measurement of TSH is easily and accurately accomplished with radioimmunoassay. The TSH level is a measure of anterior pituitary function and responsiveness to feedback inhibition in the HPT axis (7). If the circulating levels of T4 and T3 decrease, the sensitivity of the pituitary thyrotropes to TRH is increased and TSH is released in an increment related to the individual's prior point of homeostasis. TSH causes stimulation of the thyroid gland in an attempt to return its production to the prior normal range. If the thyroid fails to respond completely, this cycle continues until production is adequate or the reserve capacity of the gland is exhausted and hypothyroidism emerges. In the latter situation, the free T4 is decreased and the TSH level is elevated. Individuals whose thyroid gland is failing but is still able to produce a level of free T4 that is in the broad laboratory range of normal are considered by endocrinologists to have chemical hypothyroidism. In clinical parlance this tends to be a euphemism for trivial disease from the doctor's standpoint. Typically these patients have slightly elevated TSH levels (normal is 1 to 7 μIU/ml) and few systemic symptoms of myxedema. Nevertheless, many of these patients who have complaints of mental depression or a subjective sense of cognitive inefficiency present to psychiatrists. Although chemical hypothyroidism may seem trivial to the internist concerned with gross physical illness, its presence may be very important to the clinician interested in affective illness. Since the TSH level is always increased in primary hypothyroidism and rarely elevated by other conditions, it may actually be a better screening test for hypothyroidism for the psychiatric patient than measurement of T4 and T3RU.

TRH Stimulation Test

The TRH stimulation test is a provocative or dynamic test of the HPT axis at the level of the pituitary gland (7). Essentially this test measures the sensitivity of the anterior pituitary thyrotropes to the effects of TRH. Like the TSH level, this test is a measure of the feedback effect of the circulating hormones on the pituitary. It more directly tests TRH receptor sensitivity, however, and is able to detect alterations in the HPT axis at a time when TSH levels may still be within the laboratory range of normal (8). This test involves the administration of 500 μg of TRH intravenously after a baseline serum TSH level is obtained. Subsequently TSH is also sampled at 15, 30, 60, and sometimes 90 minutes after the injection (Figure 2). In normal control subjects, the level of TSH increases to a peak value usually at 30 minutes postinjection. When the baseline value is subtracted from the peak TSH value, one obtains a value called the delta TSH score. In normal individuals one finds delta scores from 5 to 20. In hypothyroid patients the delta score is markedly increased and values in excess of 30 are common. As the HPT axis progressively fails, first one will see an abnormally large TSH response to TRH, then an increase in serum TSH, and finally a fall in the level of the circulating hormones below the normal laboratory range. Even when the T4, T3RU, and TSH are within the normal laboratory range, an increased delta score means that the pituitary receptors have adjusted to increase their TSH response to TRH because of some change in the HPT equilibrium toward hypothyroidism. Although even baseline TSH levels are still in the normal range, the anterior pituitary has become exceptionally responsive to TRH stimulation at a time of relatively reduced circulating thyroid hormone.

THYROID ANTIBODIES

Although not a direct measure of thyroid function, screening for antibodies against thyroid tissue may be useful in the evaluation of suspected thyroid illness. Autoimmune thyroiditis is the most common cause of hypothyroidism. This illness is much more common in women and has a slowly progressive course that usually begins in early to middle adulthood. Serum can be tested for the presence of antibodies to two common antigens: thyroid microsomes and thyroglobulin. The presence of antibodies to either of these is abnormal and can be easily detected (9). High titers of antimicrosomal or antithyroglobulin antibodies are strongly suggestive of active thyroiditis, particularly in the setting of abnormal thyroid function tests.

---

1. Patients take nothing by mouth after midnight and are at rest in bed by 8:30 A.M.

2. Indwelling venous catheter is placed and a normal saline drip started to keep the line open.

3. At 8:59 A.M. blood is taken through a three-way stopcock for determination of T3RU, T3RIA, T4, and TSH levels.

4. At 9 A.M. 500 μg of TRH (protirelin) is slowly given i.v. over a 30-second period. Side effects from the infusion may include a transient sensation of warmth, desire to urinate, nausea, metallic taste, headache, dry mouth, chest tightness, or a pleasant genital sensation. These effects are generally short lived and mild.

5. Blood samples are taken through the stopcock before the TRH is administered and at 15, 30, 60, and 90 minutes after the infusion to measure changes in TSH.

Figure 2.   TRH Test Protocol

The presence of antimicrosomal antibodies has been related to thyroid disease as measured by pathological studies showing lymphocytic infiltration of the thyroid gland and elevated TSH levels (10).

HYPOTHYROIDISM AND DEPRESSION

It has long been recognized that many signs and symptoms of thyroid illness overlap with those of major depressive disorder (Figure 3). These include dysphoric mood, decreased energy and weakness, impaired cognitive ability and efficiency, anhedonia, and other neurovegetative problems. Because both depression and hypothyroidism are disorders that are associated with effective although different therapies, it is obviously important to diagnose each accurately. Psychiatric diagnostic systems such as the Research Diagnostic Criteria (RDC) (11) and the *Diagnostic and Statistical Manual of Mental Disorders*, third Edition (DSM-III) (12) emphasize careful differential diagnosis among the psychiatric syndromes and stress the importance of excluding organic etiologies. Yet it is clear that laboratory testing has an important role in the diagnostic process because there is a

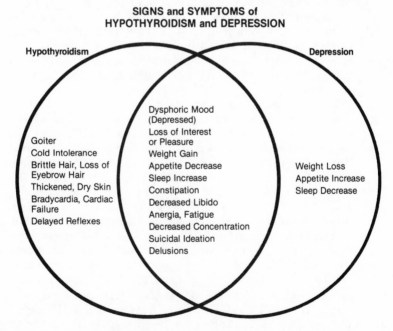

Figure 3. Signs and Symptoms of Hypothyroidism and Depression

wide overlap between the signs and symptoms of these two disorders. Screening tests for thyroid illness are most likely to be limited to the measurement of T4 and T3RU when the possibility of this diagnosis is considered. As should be apparent from earlier sections of this chapter, these tests will certainly detect patients with advanced hypothyroidism but may not identify milder degrees of the illness. Interestingly, depression is not the only medical disorder that has been recognized as a clinical variant presentation of early hypothyroidism. Anemia, coagulopathy, myopathy, and inflammatory arthritis have all been described as due to autoimmune thyroiditis at a stage when T4 and T3RU values were normal and the myxedema syndrome was absent (13). These patients did, however, have abnormal TSH levels and TRH tests. Thus it has been increasingly recognized that there is a spectrum of emerging thyroid dysfunction and a system has been created to divide this spectrum into three grades (1, 2).

Grade one or overt hypothyroidism is characterized by the classic picture of myxedema and completely abnormal laboratory findings: decreased T4, increased TSH, and an exaggerated TRH stimulation test response. Grade two or mild hypothyroidism is associated with fewer clinical symptoms and a normal T4, but an increased baseline TSH and an exaggerated TRH stimulation test response. Grade three or subclinical hypothyroidism is without any obvious "thyroid" symptoms other than depression or decreased energy. T4 and TSH levels are normal but the TRH stimulation test shows an exaggerated response.

The finding that some depressed patients manifested laboratory evidence for thyroid dysfunction when TSH levels and TRH stimulation tests were performed stimulated interest in the actual prevalence of this disorder in psychiatric patients with symptoms of depression. Initial efforts focused on hospitalized patients. In an initial study of 250 consecutive such patients, 20 (8 percent) showed some degree of hypothyroidism on comprehensive clinical evaluation and laboratory testing (14). Two patients had grade one or overt hypothyroidism with positive clinical findings and the typical laboratory findings. Eight had clinical evidence of mild hypothyroidism such as fatigue, weight gain, and dry skin along with normal T4 levels, mildly elevated TSH levels, and an increased delta score on the TRH test. Another 10 patients had no clinical symptoms of hypothyroidism other than complaints of depressed mood or lack of energy, normal T4 and TSH levels but increased TRH test scores. These findings were confirmed in another study of 270 similar patients admitted to inpatient care in hospitals in New Jersey, Georgia, and Texas (15). Of the patients in this study, 32 (12 percent) showed evidence of hypothyroidism. Of these 32 hypothyroid patients, 30 (94 percent) had either grade two or grade three hypothyroidism and would not have been detected by measurement of serum thyroxine alone.

These findings suggested that the prevalence of hypothyroidism in depressed patients was much higher than previously thought. To examine the question as to whether this finding was an artifact of the inpatient setting, outpatient studies were done. In one study of 44 consecutive outpatients meeting RDC for major unipolar depression, 6 patients (14 percent) showed laboratory evidence for either grade two or grade three hypothyroidism (16). Although this study was small, the result agrees with the inpatient studies and suggests that the increased incidence of hypothyroidism is not limited to inpatients. Furthermore it indicates that a full DSM-III syndrome can be produced by early hypothyroidism and that routine thyroid tests cannot exclude the possibility of organic dysfunction as required by the DSM-III. "Routine" thyroid testing would have only identified less than 10 percent of these patients. Taken together these studies also make it clear that thyroid dysfunction is by far the most likely condition to present as depression to the psychiatrist.

In a study recently reported by our group (29), of 156 patients who were admitted to a psychiatric inpatient service, 22 (14 percent) showed evidence of some degree of hypothyroidism. Of these patients, 16 were diagnosed as having an affective disorder rather than other psychiatric diagnoses ($\chi^2 = 8.43, p < .01$). Those depressed patients with hypothyroidism had a mean age of 39 years; 81 percent were women. Among the patients with major depression in the entire sample, there were no significant differences in symptom profiles, Carroll Rating Scale scores, or Hamilton Rating Scale for Depression scores between the euthyroid and the hypothyroid subgroups. These findings were also true for the patients with nonmajor depression. The only clinical feature that stood out in this study other than the predominance of female patients in the hypothyroid subgroup was the finding that one-third of the hypothyroid patients with depression had a positive family history of thyroid disorder. This was most frequently seen in a first-degree female relative.

The etiology of primary hypothyroidism is diverse but autoimmune illness is currently considered the most common cause. Other causes include lithium therapy, prior thyroid surgery or radioactive ablation, and discontinuation of previously prescribed thyroid hormone. Another study of 100 inpatients that identified 15 patients with evidence of hypothyroidism included screening for antithyroid antibodies (17). Of these patients, 9 (60 percent) had significant titers of antimicrosomal antibodies, suggesting active autoimmune thyroiditis. In patients without other evidence of thyroid disease, the term "symptomless autoimmune thyroiditis" has been proposed for persons with increased TSH responses to TRH infusion and circulating antithyroid antibodies (18–20). However, emerging thyroid dysfunction that is symptomless to the internist looking for gross physical dysfunction may appear as depression if a detailed psychiatric interview is accomplished.

The question that remains for research is that of therapeutics. Certainly those few grade one patients that present to psychiatrists should be treated with complete thyroid replacement. Patients with grade two or three hypothyroidism tend to be poor responders to antidepressants alone and actually seem to worsen on them because these patients are sensitive to sedative and anticholinergic side effects of these medications. They do tend to convert to responders when thyroid hormone replacement or T3 potentiation is added to the antidepressant program (21).

Treatment alternatives for these patients have not yet been studied in double-blind fashion. It is felt that primary hypothyroidism is a progressive illness. There are some reports that patients with mild hypothyroidism are at increased risk for cardiac disease and myocardial dysfunction. There are also proven beneficial cardiac responses to thyroid replacement in patients with grade two hypothyroidism. It is also true, somewhat ironically, that many internists treating patients with thyroid replacement for overt hypothyroidism require the laboratory normalization of TSH levels or the TRH stimulation test (22, 23). While a patient who presents with grade two or chemical hypothyroidism and few clinical symptoms may not be felt to warrant thyroid replacement, a grade one or overt patient may not be considered adequately treated if thyroid replacement still leaves the patient with the laboratory profile of either the grade two or three patient. However, a recent double-blind, placebo-controlled study of nondepressed patients with grade two hypothyroidism did show that T4 replacement was beneficial in terms of improving mild clinical symptoms and improving objective measures of cardiac function (30). It is also likely that many grade two and three patients with psychiatric symptoms will respond well to thyroid replacement alone, although this has not been proven in large studies. In a small open study (15), 8 of 10 patients with grade two or three hypothyroidism who met RDC for either major or minor depression responded to thyroid replacement alone over a period of 1 month. After a year follow-up period, only one of the responders had relapsed and that patient was the only patient in the study that had an abnormal dexamethasone suppression test (suggesting concurrent major depressive disorder) at the time of initial evaluation. That patient subsequently responded to the addition of an antidepressant to the thyroid replacement program. In another open study (29), 9 patients with grade two hypothyroidism and either major or minor depression were followed for 6 months on an average daily dose of 100 μg of T4. Patients were given enough thyroid replacement to suppress their baseline TSH levels below 4.0 μIU/ml and were judged recovered if their Carroll Rating Scale and Hamilton Rating Scale for Depression scores both dropped below 10 from pretreatment means of 23.4 and 18.6, respectively. During the treatment period, 2 of 5 patients with major depression and all 4 patients with nonmajor depression responded. The 3 remaining patients with major depression subsequently responded to the addition of either electroconvulsive therapy or tricyclic antidepressants. All 3 of these patients had previously failed to respond to antidepressants alone. There have been no double-blind, placebo-controlled studies of depressed patients with grade two or three hypothyroidism yet reported.

Nevertheless, given the proven medical benefits, initial treatment with thyroid hormone is recommended for all grade two patients with the addition of antidepressants if the response in terms of mood and energy is weak after 2 months. The treatment of grade three patients is less certain and should be individualized. Certainly an adjunctive trial of thyroid replacement should be considered if the patient has not responded to prior treatment with antidepressants; grade three patients are particularly responsive to T3 potentiation (21). Thyroid replacement should be enough to return TSH and TRH values into the normal laboratory range (23). For most individuals this is accomplished with an eventual dose of 75 to 150 μg of T4 daily. Elderly patients should be advanced more slowly than younger patients and seldom require more than 100 μg daily (23). All grade three patients who are not treated with thyroid replacement should be closely followed for the possibility of progressive thyroid failure, especially if they are treated with medications such as lithium.

It should be appreciated that the finding that early thyroid failure is the most common medical condition to mimic depression is probably not a chance phenomenon. Whybrow and Prange (24) have hypothesized a close relationship between thyroid function and the responsiveness of central catecholamine receptors. Thyroid hormones increase beta-adrenergic receptor sensitivity, and noradrenergic activity would therefore be enhanced or diminished by corresponding levels of thyroid in the central nervous system. Following the classic biogenic theory of depression, either a thyroid deficit or a neurotransmitter deficit would be expressed the same as decreased effective beta-adrenergic activity and clinical depression (25).

CASE REPORT

Ms. A., a 27-year-old female executive, was referred to the hospital from the intensive care unit of a general hospital following an overdose of amitriptyline. This was the second overdose of an antidepressant in a period of 6 months. Ms. A. had been in psychotherapy with a psychologist for 12 months prior to this admission and had been followed concurrently by a psychiatrist for 9 months for purposes of medication provision. Her chief complaint was "I tried to commit suicide twice and I guess that means that I am depressed." She had no prior history of psychiatric hospitalization nor was there any family history of affective disorder. The patient complained of depressed mood, decreased energy, increased need for sleep (which seemed to worsen following administration of amitriptyline), anhedonia, impaired concentration and memory, progressive feelings of hopelessness, and a desire to withdraw socially. At the time of admission the patient expressed a feeling of disappointment that her second suicide attempt had been unsuccessful and stated that she would probably try again to kill herself. Her Beck Depression Inventory score was 28; Hamilton Rating Scale for Depression was 22. General physical examination was within normal limits. General medical screening tests were also normal. The T4 was 6.5 (normal, 4–12); the T3RU was 26.0 (normal, 24–36); the FTI was 5.6 (normal, 4–12); the TSH level was 4.8 (normal, 1–7). A TRH stimulation test revealed a delta score of 27.1 (normal, 5–20). Antithyroid antibodies were not present. A 6-point dexamethasone suppression test showed normal suppression at all time points. The patient was diagnosed as having grade three hypothyroidism and it was elected to treat her with thyroid replacement alone, especially since she had not tolerated antidepressants and had also used them destructively. After 1 month the patient was markedly improved on thyroid replacement alone. The Beck Depression Inventory score was 3 and the Hamilton Rating Scale for Depression score was 2. The T4 was 11.2, the T3RU was 28.8, and the TSH was less than 1. Following discharge from the hospital, the patient has continued to take sodium T4 (Synthroid) 125 µg daily for a follow-up period of 2.5 years. She has not received any other medications. The patient has remained free of depression and anergia and has continued to be productive in her professional and personal life.

THYROID WORK-UP

Clearly the practicing clinician must screen all patients for physical illness. Not only is this consistent with the role of the psychiatrist as a physician but also many authors have pointed out the high percentage of patients with physical disorders either causing or contributing to the clinical problem for which psychiatric care is sought (26–28). In evaluating patients with suspected thyroid disease, the clinician needs to rely on history, physical examination, and laboratory testing. The fact that the patient has a full depressive syndrome does not exclude secondary depression, particularly in the case of thyroid disorder. All patients presenting with lack of energy and depression should have measurement of T4, T3RU, and TSH. This panel of tests will pick up all patients with overt and mild hypothyroidism. One-third of patients in the above-described studies would have been detected with this panel. Patients who are still suspected to have subclinical hypothyroidism on the basis of family history of thyroid disorder, female sex, failure to respond to or intolerance of antidepressants, and perhaps depression of the severity to require inpatient care should have a TRH infusion test. If that test score is abnormally increased, antithyroid antibodies should also be measured.

REFERENCES

1. Evered DC, Ormston BJ, Smith PA, et al: Grades of hypothyroidism. Br Med J 1:657–662, 1973

2. Bastenie PA, Bonnyns M, Vanhaelst L: Grades of subclinical hypothyroidism in asymptomatic autoimmune thyroiditis revealed by the Thyrotropin-Releasing-Hormone Test. J Clin Endocrinol Metab 51:163–166, 1980

3. Martin JB, Reichlin S, Brown GM: Clinical Neuroendocrinology. Philadelphia, FA Davis Co, 1977

4. Jackson IM: Thyrotropin-releasing hormone. N Engl J Med 306:145, 1982

5. Morley JE: Neuroendocrine control of thyrotropin secretion. Endocr Rev 2(4):296, 1981

6. Blum M: Easier understanding of the new thyroid tests. Resident and Staff Physicians 27:72–90, 1981

7. Ormston BJ, Garry R, Cryer RJ, et al: Thyrotropin-releasing hormone as a thyroid function test. Lancet 2:10–14, 1971

8. Sternbach H, Gener RH, Gwirstman HE: the Thyrotropin-Releasing-Hormone Stimulation Test: a review. J Clin Psychiatry 43:1,4, 1982

9. Fink JN, Beall GN: Immunological aspects of endocrine disease. JAMA 248:2696–2700, 1982

10. Hawkins BR, Dawkins RL, Burger HG, et al: Diagnostic significance of thyroid microsomal antibodies in a randomly selected population. Lancet 2:1057–1059, 1980

11. Spitzer RL, Endicott J, Robins E: Research Diagnostic Criteria (RDC) for a Selected Group of Functional Disorders. New York, New York State Psychiatric Institute, 1980

12. American Psychiatric Association: Diagnostic and Statistical Manual of Mental Disorders. 3rd ed. Washington, DC, American Psychiatric Association, 1980

13. Klein I, Levey GS: Unusual manifestations of hypothyroidism. Arch Intern Med 144:123–128, 1984

14. Gold MS, Pottash ALC, Extein I: Hypothyroidism in depression: evidence from complete thyroid function evaluation. JAMA 245:1919–1922, 1981

15. Dackis CA, Goggans FC, Bloodworth R, et al: The prevalence of hypothryoidism in psychiatric populations. Presented at the Annual Meeting of the American Psychiatric Association, New York, May 1983

16. Sternbach HA, Gold MS, Pottash ALC, et al: Thyroid failure and protirelin test abnormalities in depressed outpatients. JAMA, 249:618–620, 1983

17. Gold MS, Pottash ALC, Extein I: "Symptomless" autoimmune thyroiditis in depression. Psychiatry Res 6:261–269, 1982

18. Bonnyns M, Vanhaelst L, Bastenie PA: Asymptomatic atrophic thyroiditis. Horm Res 16:338–344, 1982

19. Gordon A, Lamberg BA: Natural course of symptomless autoimmune thyroiditis. Lancet 2:1234–1238, 1975

20. Tunbridge WM, Brewis M, French JM, et al: Natural history of autoimmune thyroiditis. Br Med J 282:258, 1981

21. Targum SD, Greenberg RD, Harmon RL, et al: Thyroid hormone and the TRH Stimulation Test in refractory depression. J Clin Psychiatry 45:345–346, 1984

22. Ridgeway EC, Cooper DS, Walker H, et al: Peripheral responses to thyroid hormone before and after L-thyroxine therapy in patients with sub-clinical hypothyroidism. J Clin Endocrinol Metab 53:1238–1242, 1981

23. Davis FB, La Mantia RS, Spaulding SW, et al: Estimation of physiologic replacement dose of levothyroxine in elderly patients with hypothyroidism. Arch Intern Med 144:1752–1754, 1984

24. Whybrow BC, Prange HA: A hypothesis of thyroid-catecholamine-receptor interaction: its relevance to affective illness. Arch Gen Psychiatry 38:106–113, 1981

25. Schildkraut JJ: Catecholamine hypothesis of affective disorders: a review of supporting evidence. Am J Psychiatry 122:509–522, 1965

26. Hall RCW, Popkin NK, Devaul RA, et al: Physical illness presenting as psychiatric disease. Arch Gen Psychiatry 35:1315, 1978

27. Koranyi EK: Morbidity and rate of undiagnosed physical illness in a psychiatric clinic population. Arch Gen Psychiatry 36:414, 1979

28. Estroff TW, Gold MS: Psychiatric misdiagnosis, in Advances in Psychopharmacology: Predicting and Improving Treatment Response. Edited by Gold MS, Lydiard RB, Carman J. Boca Raton, Florida CRC Press, 1984, pp 33–66

29. Goggans FC, Allen RM, et al: Thyroid disorders in psychiatric practice. Presented at the Annual Meeting of the American Psychiatric Association, Dallas, 1985

30. Cooper DS, Halpern R, et al: L-thyroxine therapy in subclinical hypothyroidism. Ann Inter Med 101:18–24, 1984

Chapter 5

Behavioral Disturbances Associated with Disorders of the Hypothalamic-Pituitary-Adrenal System

Victor I. Reus, M.D.
Jeffrey R. Berlant, M.D.

Chapter 5

Behavioral Disturbances Associated with Disorders of the Hypothalamic-Pituitary-Adrenal System

One of the goals of differential diagnosis is to evolve a set of inclusion and exclusion criteria by which a clinician can categorize a patient's signs and symptoms and thus determine appropriate treatment and probable course of illness. Deciding which symptoms are primary, which secondary, and which are to be given greater valence than others is still a rather arbitrary process in many areas of medicine, the result being that it has been quite difficult to construct computer-based "expert" systems of diagnostic practice. It is particularly important to examine how such information is treated in the psychiatric diagnostic system because behavioral symptomatology is rarely utilized in a specific fashion by the other medical specialties in diagnostic assessment. For example, one of the main criteria of either a manic or major depressive episode according to the *Diagnostic and Statistical Manual of Mental Disorders*, Third Edition (DSM-III) (1) is that the behavioral symptomatology be "not due to any organic mental disorder." In such cases, it is suggested that the proper diagnosis is that of "Organic Affective Syndrome" (DSM-III 293.83). It is noted that the "clinical phenomenology of the syndrome is the same as that of a manic or major depressive episode" and that "endocrine disorders are another important etiologic factor, and may produce either depressive or manic syndromes. Examples are hyper- and hypothyroidism and hyper- and hypoadrenocortisolism." In discussing the differential diagnosis, DSM-III further states that "in affective disorders no specific organic factor can be demonstrated." It is clear then that in resolving the differential diagnosis, the burden exists on the clinician to decide what a "specific

113

organic factor" is and at what point a behavioral syndrome is "due" to some other associated biological phenomenon. Since many psychiatric patients can be shown to possess some degree of endocrine dysfunction, this is neither a simple nor inconsequential task. Most medical syndromes are likewise not operationally defined and may themselves exist on a continuum of severity of dysfunction. In Cushing's syndrome, for example, recognition that the syndrome can be associated with mild perturbations of hypothalamic-pituitary-adrenal (HPA) function can occur in a transient and episodic fashion, be characterized by spontaneous remission, and be unassociated with observable cushingoid stigmata would indicate that the differential diagnosis of an individual case might be problematic (Table 1).

As the French physician Laignel-Lavastine (2) noted in 1919:

> The endocrine disorders in nervous syndromes, whether they have been established by clinical or anatomical methods or induced by physiological or therapeutic proofs, are face-to-face with the nervous syndromes. . . . The frequency of pathological endocrino-psychic associations are not explicable alone by fortuitous coincidences and more or less immediate attachments. It seems to me necessary to admit, in certain cases at least, a relationship of causality. (p. 33)

Without evidence to the contrary, it is more parsimonious to regard endocrinologic changes in populations defined on behavioral grounds as pathophysiologically linked to those more severe "primary" endocrinologic disturbances, which are in turn accompanied by symptomatic changes in behavior. In such circumstances, current algorithms of differential diagnosis may be based on historical or statistical rather than physiological principles. It is difficult, therefore, to proclaim a clear differentiation between medical and psychiatric disorders in cases where the mechanism of behavioral dysfunction is unknown. In light of these considerations, this section will review the behavioral symptomatology of primary disorders of HPA function, as well as parallel findings of HPA dysfunction in primary psychiatric populations, and discuss possible clinical and research approaches to individuals presenting with disturbances in both areas of function.

Behavioral Symptoms of Cushing's Syndrome

Whether the result of adrenal hyperplasia, pituitary adenoma, ectopic adrenocorticotropic hormone (ACTH)-producing tumor, chronic alcohol use, or intracranial pathology, Cushing's syndrome is frequently associated with a change in mental status. In general, no pathognomonic behavioral profile has been described for hypercortisolemic states, although most reports have underscored prominent

changes in affect and cognition (3–7). In a classic description provided by Cushing (8), it was noted that the patient was "without
energy, easily fatigued, unable to concentrate his mind on his work,
and fits of unnatural irritability alternated with periods of depression"
(p. 177). It is clear that Cushing himself did not regard this as a
casual observation since, in a more general review (9) 19 years earlier,
he underscored the fact that it was "quite probable that in similar
fashion a disorder primarily involving any other member of the ductless gland series leads not only to its peculiar somatic alterations but
also to an accompanying and characteristic mental change" (p. 972).
In a particularly intriguing parallel comment, he further noted that
out of 75 pituitary glands sent to him from the Worchester State
Mental Hospital, there "appeared to be no examples among them
of what might be called histologically normal glands, though certainly
many of them must have been normal within physiologic limits" (8,
p. 984). Since these original observations, most investigators have
found abnormal behavioral symptomatology in anywhere from 40
to 90 percent of Cushing's syndrome patients (3–7). Frank psychotic
symptomatology characterized by auditory and visual hallucinations,
severe confusion, paranoia, or mania is evident in 10 to 20 percent
of the cases and suicidal ideation or action is common. In general,
euphoria and increased motoric activity are observed early in the
course of illness, with depression, insomnia, fatigue, loss of libido,
emotional lability, and cognitive impairment more pronounced in
later stages.

Unfortunately most reports of behavioral symptomatology in
Cushing's syndrome have been uncontrolled, retrospective, and selective in nature. Since most studies do not distinguish patients with
Cushing's disease from those with Cushing's syndrome, this review
will use the term "Cushing's syndrome" in the most general sense,
including patients with pituitary pathology. Several recent studies
have attempted to control for these variables. In a consecutive unselected series of 29 patients, Cohen (10) found that 86 percent of
the patients were significantly depressed and that there was a family
history of depression or suicide in half of the cases. He further noted
that depression was rapidly relieved when the hypercortisolemia was
successfully treated. Supporting an intriguing observation made originally by Hurxthal and O'Sullivan (11), a significant percentage of
the patient population reported that the onset of somatic symptomatology had been preceded by a period of extreme psychological
stress. Whether this sequence of events is related to serendipity,
causation, or reflective of an underlying subclinical endocrinopathy
is unclear, although it is evident that changes in the mental state may

Table 1. Problems in the Differential Diagnosis of Cushing's Syndrome and Primary Affective Disorder

	Cushing's Syndrome	Affective Disorder (Representative Study)
Secretion rate	Increased	May be increased
DST response (low dose)	Nonsuppression	Possible nonsuppression
DST response (high dose)	Possible nonsuppression	Possible nonsuppression (36)
Cortisol response to hypoglycemia	Blunted	May be blunted
Plasma ACTH level postdexamethasone	May be increased	May be increased (34)
ACTH response to cortisol	May be altered	May be altered (34,35)
Response to metyrapone	May be increased	May be increased (33)
	May improve mood	Mood effects unknown
Circadian variation in plasma cortisol	Blunted but may be normal	May be blunted
CSF CRF level	Unknown	May be increased

Response to CRF	May be augmented	May be blunted (39)
Physical signs of hypocortisolemia	May be absent (28) Nonspecific (23)	May be present (29, 58)
Sleep architecture	↓ delta sleep	↓ delta sleep (4)
Affective symptomatology	Frequently present	Present
Course of illness (behavioral and hormonal)	May be cyclic or episodic	May be cyclic
Family history of affective illness	May be present (10)	May be absent
Pituitary microadenoma	Frequently present	Frequency unknown
Response to cyproheptadine	May decrease hypercortisolemia (51)	May alter mood (59)
Response to tricyclic antidepressants	Unknown	May alter mood and HPA function
Response to lithium	Unknown	Lowers cortisol level (66) and prevents steroid psychosis (65)

be the earliest and most prominent presenting features. In a controlled study by Kelly et al. (12), it was noted that patients with active Cushing's syndrome were significantly more depressed by Hamilton rating scores than patients who had been successfully treated or patients with other pituitary tumors. Correction of the Cushing's syndrome alleviated the associated depression (13). In a more detailed prospective study (14), increased levels of cortisol and ACTH were associated with increased impairment in affect, decreased concentration and memory, decreased libido, and insomnia. One-third of the patients had moderate to marked deficits in language and nonlanguage tests of higher cortical function, as well as additional impairments in sensory and motor function, particularly evident in tasks involving visual processing (15, 16).

HPA Dysfunction in Psychiatric Illness

A preponderance of evidence has indicated that disturbances in glucocorticoid regulation are a common feature of many psychiatric syndromes. These biologic changes are observed most frequently in depressed patients, but have also been reported in patients with eating disorders, panic disorder, mania, borderline disorder, Alzheimer's dementia, obsessive-compulsive disorder, and schizoaffective disorder (17). In the majority of studies, a decreased suppression of cortisol in response to dexamethasone is evident. In patients with major depressive disorder, increases in plasma, urine, and cerebrospinal fluid (CSF) levels of cortisol have also been demonstrated. Other studies have shown evidence for increased cortisol secretion, an attenuated circadian rhythm in corticotropin and cortisol secretion, increased adrenal sensitivity, increased insulin resistance and a blunted cortisol response to hypoglycemia, increased corticotropin secretion, and, most recently, a blunted corticotropin response to the infusion of ovine corticotropin-releasing factor (CRF). It has been suggested accordingly that the primary defect in regulation leading to these phenomena is at the level of the hypothalamus or limbic system. In depressed patients, a hypersecretion of CRF is hypothesized, with subsequent down-regulation of pituitary corticotrophs. It might be expected that plasma corticotropin levels would be either normal or increased, depending on the pattern and duration of hypothalamic stimulation, the pituitary reserve available, and the compensatory increases in corticotropin formation and storage. Changes in adrenal sensitivity may contribute to findings of elevation in cortisol level and be secondary either to alterations in corticotropin secretion or to the direct effects of CRF on adrenal receptors.

Even though the pattern of changes in HPA regulation is becoming better delineated, how such changes come into being and what their relationship is to behavioral symptomatology is still unclear. On the basis of data derived from animal studies, a number of hypotheses can be constructed. From one perspective, the neuroendocrine changes observed may derive from a genetically mediated alteration, possibly involving the regulation of a "parent" compound, pro-opiomelanocortin. Alternatively, it is possible that such alterations in neuroendocrine "tuning" derive from physiologic or environmental influences on critical time locked neuroendocrine encoding periods during early development. To the extent that neuroendocrine systems respond and adapt to recurrent stress demand, the phenomena observed may in some cases be ascribable to, or affected by, stressful life events in adulthood. In a subgroup of depressed individuals, as in Cushing's patients, microadenomas may be responsible. In actuality all these factors are likely to contribute to the array of HPA disturbances described and possibly to the behavioral phenomenology as well. In a number of behavioral syndromes, the dysfunction observed might be better conceptualized as a disorder of homeostatic regulation rather than reflective of a disease process per se. To this end, there is increasing evidence that patients exhibiting HPA dysfunction commonly have an associated increase in noradrenergic sympathetic output (18). In such individuals there may be evidence that the behavioral dysfunction that occurs is commonly stress induced or precipitated, stress in these terms being defined broadly to include such things as the physiologic demands of seasonal change, as well as psychologically stressful events. The behavioral correlates of disturbances in HPA regulation are still relatively unexplored, although some preliminary evidence would indicate that symptoms of depression, anxiety, and cognitive disturbance are prominent (19, 20).

Difficulties in Differential Diagnosis

Cushing's original descriptions of presumptive basophil hyperpituitarism were characterized by profound painful obesity, hypertrichosis, osteoporosis, hypertension, and sexual dysfunction. It has since become clear that such signs are neither inevitably found nor specific to individuals who meet laboratory requirements for the diagnosis of Cushing's syndrome. Fewer than half of the cases diagnosed according to laboratory standards present with classic features, while the features themselves occur in high prevalence in the general population (21–24). Is it always possible, then, to distinguish a psychiatric patient presenting with signs of HPA dysfunction from a patient with "Cushing's syndrome"?

Traditionally, one of the foremost considerations in such an assessment was the presence or absence of physical stigmata of hyper-cortisolemia. Increasingly, however, it is recognized that classic examples of chronic tissue exposure to elevated glucocorticoid level are rare and that a number of cases of Cushing's syndrome are almost asymptomatic. Documented cases of hypercortisolism presenting only with osteoporosis (25), hypokalemic alkalosis (26), short stature (27), or mild obesity (28) have been reported. The report by Saad et al. (28), confirmed by tissue pathology, is of particular interest because their patient presented with acute psychosis and cognitive impairment in the *absence* of characteristic clinical stigmata of the illness. In addition, the patient was noted to have normal plasma cortisol levels and perfect diurnal rhythm on several days of assessment. Claims that psychiatric patients with hypercortisolemia do not show cushingoid stigmata and that the HPA dysfunction in these cases is state dependent are thus somewhat beside the point. Empirical investigation of the prevalence of such signs and symptoms in psychiatric patients presenting with HPA disturbance are, in fact, lacking. In a recent study, however, a subgroup of such patients showed changes in hematologic indices consistent with those observed in Cushing's syndrome and statistically different from psychiatric patients without evidence of HPA disturbance (29). The relative rarity of the more profound stigmata, such as "buffalo hump," may be secondary to lesser degrees of HPA dysregulation, decreased tissue exposure over time, or a deficit in glucocorticoid receptor mechanisms. Some indirect evidence for the latter hypothesis has recently been presented, and a primary disorder of cortisol resistance has been identified in humans, although its relationship to behavioral dysfunction is unknown (30, 31).

Nearly all of the HPA abnormalities described in Cushing's syndrome can occur in patients with primary psychiatric disorder. As noted, these include increased plasma and CSF levels of cortisol, increased cortisol excretion, increased nocturnal episodes of cortisol release, increased plasma ACTH, and decreased circadian variation of cortisol release (17, 32, 33). Alterations in ACTH and cortisol response to cortisol infusion have also been reported in both primary endocrine and psychiatric populations (34, 35). Several authors have suggested that cortisol response to insulin-induced hypoglycemia and cortisol response to high-dose dexamethasone administration might reliably be used to differentiate those patients indistinguishable on other grounds (24). These recommendations, however, ignore other data that clearly indicate that abnormal responses may be found in psychiatric patients in these tests as well (36–38). One recent investigation utilizing an ovine CRF infusion has indicated that this test may be useful in the differential diagnosis. Some patients with depression were found to have a blunted ACTH response to CRF in comparison with Cushing's syndrome patients who had augmented responses (39). While some psychiatric patients may have abnormal results on such neuroendocrine assessments of HPA function, patients with Cushing's syndrome may in turn have relatively normal responses. In one recent article, for example, two women with typical Cushing's disease were found to have a normal variation in serum cortisol concentration (40).

Assessment of course of illness likewise may be unhelpful in differentiating between these patient groups. Cyclic and episodic variants of Cushing's syndrome are increasingly recognized, although undoubtedly still underdiagnosed because of assessments performed in well periods and because tissue exposure to hypercortisolemia may be too short to produce definitive somatic stigmata. In parallel to the well-described cyclicity of affective disorders, patients with cyclic Cushing's syndrome can have rhythmic fluctuations of ACTH and cortisol secretion ranging from 2 to as long as 88 days (41–44). In a number of such cases, alterations in mental state were closely linked to changes in HPA function, as has been described for patients with major depression. In two reports, the patient appeared to exhibit changes in mood consistent with bipolar affective disorder in association with cyclic variations of "transient" Cushing's syndrome (45, 46).

Spontaneous remissions occur in patients with Cushing's syndrome, presumably those exhibiting periodic hormonogenesis. The cause of the hypercortisolism in these cases described is frequently an abdominal or pituitary tumor, although an association with an empty sella turcica has also been described (47). Emotional lability was a prominent presenting feature in this latter report. One subjective impression that might be derived in a review of this literature is that changes in mood and mental state are noted more consistently in descriptions of "intermittent," "transient," or "periodic" Cushing's syndrome. This seems particularly true in situations in which the locus of hormonal dysfunction is thought to be hypothalamic or diencephalic (3, 48, 49).

Radiologic evaluation is usually not helpful in the differential diagnosis. Although as many as 80 percent of patients with Cushing's syndrome are found to have pituitary adenomas or areas of marked hyperplasia at surgery, these are usually too small to be reliably identified with current radiologic techniques.

THERAPEUTIC CONSIDERATIONS

One of the principal goals to be achieved in the differential diagnosis is the formulation of a treatment plan that is optimally therapeutic for the specified condition. This is a particularly important consideration with the population under discussion since the mode of intervention in the one condition is usually surgical while in the other it is pharmacological. The principal goal of treatment of Cushing's syndrome is, of course, correction of the hypercortisolemia. Since approximately 60 to 80 percent of all patients with Cushing's syndrome are found to have basophilic microadenomas of the pituitary, transphenoidal microadenectomy has emerged as one of the principal approaches to reduction of hypercortisolism, despite variance in the long-term efficacy of this procedure among centers (50, 51). Partial response and relapse are not infrequent, and some investigators view morphologic pituitary changes as secondary to increased hypothalamic drive (51). Radiation of the pituitary, using cobalt radiotherapy and proton beam techniques, has also been used with efficacy in a number of cases. In general, the majority of Cushing's syndrome patients with behavioral pathology experience an improvement in mental status in association with reduction of hypercortisolism. In certain cases, however, neither reduction in hypercortisolism nor improvement in mental status is observed following pituitary surgery, leaving moot the issue of diagnosis and etiology (24).

Unfortunately, the prevalence of pituitary microadenomas in a psychiatric population selected on the basis of some index of HPA dysfunction is unknown. Two classic studies of general psychiatric populations by Cushing and Laignel-Lavastine reported gross evidence of pituitary pathology while several recent autopsy series of unselected patients not known to have pituitary disease prior to death have found a prevalence of microadenomas of the pituitary ranging from 10 to 27 percent (51, 52). In a population selected on the basis of endocrine dysfunction, it might be expected that the prevalence would be even greater. These findings suggest that the existence of a pituitary microadenoma upon surgical exploration cannot be used post hoc to distinguish the primary endocrinologic and primary psychiatric populations described, since in a number of cases such pathologic tissue changes neither result in chronic or progressive symptomatology, nor are they invariably associated with endocrine dysfunction.

Several pharmacologic treatments have been used with success in the reduction of hypercortisolemia and, concomitantly, in improvement of behavioral symptomatology. Cyproheptadine, a serotonergic and histaminergic antagonist, has been perhaps the most widely used agent. Bromocriptine and sodium valproate have also been used with success (51, 54–57). Since hypercortisolemia seems intrinsically linked to behavioral pathology in Cushing's disease, the question emerges as to whether these drugs have concomitant mood-altering effects in psychiatric patients, particularly those with signs of HPA dysregulation. A few studies indicate that this may be the case. In one report, cyproheptadine had both mood-altering and somatic effects in a patient with bipolar affective illness *and* cushingoid features (58), whereas in another the drug appeared to trigger a hypomanic episode in a woman with documented bipolar affective disorder (59). Preliminary evidence that cyproheptadine might be useful in the treatment of anorexia nervosa, both in terms of improvement in mood and in weight gain, is of particular interest because of the HPA changes in this syndrome and possible pathophysiologic associations with Cushing's syndrome (60). Both bromocriptine and sodium valproate have significant effects on mood, although whether these effects are associated with concomitant change in HPA function is not known.

There has been no controlled investigation of the effects of traditional psychiatric treatments either on the behavioral symptomatology or the hypercortisolism associated with Cushing's syndrome. In clinical reports, electroconvulsive therapy (ECT) has been used successfully in the treatment of depression associated with hyperparathyroid and HPA disorders (61, 62). ECT has also been noted to result in a progressive lowering of postdexamethasone cortisol values in parallel with an improvement in mood (63). Reports on the efficacy of tricyclic and monoamine oxidase inhibitor antidepressant treatment of depressive symptomatology and hypercortisolemia in Cushing's syndrome are lacking. There is evidence, however, that lithium carbonate may prevent iatrogenic corticosteroid psychosis (64, 65). Recent data documenting a decrease in cortisol levels in association with lithium therapy, together with evidence that cortisol production is sensitive to the influence of a number of psychoactive agents, might indicate that these agents could be used with success in the treatment of endocrine dysfunction in some patients with Cushing's syndrome (13). In one classic case involving periodic hypothalamic discharge and interpreted as representing a case of "periodic" Cushing's syndrome, the principal effective agent was chlorpromazine (45).

A logical extrapolation of this line of inquiry would be to question whether traditional approaches to the hypercortisolemia in Cushing's syndrome might not also be used with success in the treatment of psychiatric patients with HPA dysfunction. The psychopharmacologic properties of such agents as trilostane, aminoglutethimide, or proposed CRF antagonists might be worthy of specific investigation, although concerns about toxicity would be relevant.

DISCUSSION

In cases where the classic symptom profile and history are present, the diagnosis of Cushing's syndrome should not be problematic, although the proper selection of treatment stratagem may be complicated and controversial. In many medical syndromes, however, the classic presentation is a rare entity reserved for medical textbooks and grand rounds presentations. Medical conditions defined on operational laboratory criteria can present with varying degrees of symptomatology. These illness states need not be progressive in nature nor associated with the same degree of risk. Hypercholesterolemia and hyperglycemia are useful examples. Profound and prolonged elevations in these substances are associated with characteristic changes in target tissues, but the predictive and diagnostic utility of moderate degrees of elevation is less clear. If some patients with Cushing's syndrome fall on a continuum with patients with "primary" affective disorder and HPA dysfunction, traditional approaches to diagnosis and treatment in both endocrinology and psychiatry might profitably be reexamined.

For a significant number of patients, particularly those with more modest degrees of neuroendocrine dysfunction, the diagnosis and treatment received may today depend more on the initial and motivating symptomatology than on the full characteristics of the illness process itself. The symptomatology that is of specific interest to a given specialty tends to receive the greatest investigation and attention, while other possibly connected aspects of the symptom complex are either ignored or viewed as unrelated or secondary in nature. Thus, studies of patients with Cushing's disease in the endocrinologic literature only rarely make mention of behavioral function and usually in an unquantified manner, while studies of dexamethasone "nonsuppressors" in the psychiatric literature fail to provide concomitant assessments of menstrual cycle, blood pressure, glucose regulation, or weight.

A similar overlap in patient populations and consequent conflict in diagnostic and treatment practices may exist with patients who present with associated symptoms of anxiety and hypertension. Unfortunately, as long as official diagnostic practice in psychiatry requires the exclusion of organic etiology for the diagnosis of major psychiatric syndromes, it is unlikely that any formal integration of such interactions between biological and behavioral function will occur. Construction of multivariate matrices of a variety of quantified signs and symptoms, possible with current computer technology, may more adequately encompass the full array of dynamic and interrelated illness data and result in more logical and useful clinical classifications than currently exist.

REFERENCES

1. American Psychiatric Association: Diagnostic and Statistical Manual of Mental Disorders. 3rd ed. Washington, DC, American Psychiatric Association, 1980

2. Laignel-Lavastine M: The Internal Secretions and the Nervous System. New York, Nervous & Mental Disease Publishing Co, 1919

3. Carroll BJ: Psychiatric disorders and steroids, in Neuroregulators and Psychiatric Disorders. Edited by Usdin E, Hamburg DA, Barchas JD. New York, Oxford University Press, 1977

4. Pepper GM, Krieger DT: Hypothalamic-pituitary-adrenal abnormalities in depression: their possible relation to central mechanisms regulating ACTH release, in Neurobiology of Mood Disorders. Edited by Post R, Ballenger J. Baltimore, Williams & Wilkins, 1984

5. Gifford S, Gunderson JG: Cushing's disease as a psychosomatic disorder: a report of 10 cases. Medicine 49:397–409, 1970

6. Whitlock FA: Symptomatic Affective Disorders: A Study of Depression and Mania Associated with Physical Disease and Medication. New York, Academic Press, 1982

7. Cohen LM, Molitch ME: Psychiatric aspects of pituitary tumors, in Psychiatric Medicine Update: Massachusetts General Hospital Reviews for Physicians. Edited by Manschrech TC, Murray GB. New York, Elsevier, 1984

8. Cushing H: The basophil adenomas of the pituitary body and their clinical manifestations (pituitary basophilism). Bulletin of the Johns Hopkins Hospital L:137–195, 1932

9. Cushing H: Psychic disturbances associated with disorders of the ductless glands. American Journal of Insanity 69:965–990, 1913

10. Cohen SI: Cushing's syndrome: a psychiatric study of 29 patients. Br J Psychiatry 136:120–124, 1980

11. Hurxthal C, O'Sullivan S: Cushing's syndrome: clinical differential diagnosis and complications. Ann Intern Med 51:1–16, 1959

12. Kelly WF, Checkley SA, Bender DA: Cushing's syndrome, tryptophan and depression. Br J Psychiatry 136:125–132, 1980

13. Kelly WF, Checkley SA, Bender DA, et al: Cushing's syndrome and depression: a prospective study of 26 patients. Br J Psychiatry 142:16–19, 1983

14. Whelan TB, Schteingart DE, Starkman MN, et al: Neuropsychological deficits in Cushing's syndrome. J Nerv Ment Dis 168:753–757, 1980

15. Starkman MN, Schteingart DE, Schork MA: Depressed mood and other psychiatric manifestations of Cushing's syndrome: relationship to hormone levels. Psychosom Med 43:3–18, 1981

16. Starkman MN, Schteingart DE: Neuropsychiatric manifestations of patients with Cushing's syndrome: relationship to cortisol and adrenocorticotropic hormone levels. Arch Intern Med 141:215–219, 1981

17. Reus VI: Toward an understanding of cortisol dysregulation in major depression: a review of studies of the dexamethasone suppression test and urinary free cortisol. Psychiatric Medicine 3:1–21, 1985

18. Jimerson DC, Insel TR, Reus VI, et al: Increased plasma MHPG in dexamethasone-resistant depressed patients. Arch Gen Psychiatry 40:173–176, 1983

19. Reus VI: Pituitary-adrenal disinhibition as the independent variable in the assessment of behavioral symptoms. Biol Psychiatry 17:317–326, 1982

20. Reus VI: Hormonal mediation of the memory disorder in depression. Drug Development Research 4:489–500, 1984

21. Reus VI: Diagnosis and treatment in endocrinology and psychiatry: from Cushing's syndrome to disorders of mood, in Emotions in Health and Illness: Applications to Clinical Practice. Edited by Van Dyke C, Temoshok L, Zegans LS. New York, Grune & Stratton, 1984

22. Burke CW: Disorders of the cortisol productions (1), in Adrenal Cortex in Practical Medicine. London, Gray-Mills, 1973

23. Ross EJ, Linch DC: Cushing's syndrome—killing disease: discriminatory value of signs and symptoms aiding early diagnosis. Lancet 2:646–649, 1982

24. Aron DC, Tyrrell JB, Fitzgerald PA, et al: Cushing's syndrome: problems in diagnosis. Medicine 60:25–35, 1981

25. Hough S, Teitelbaum SL, Bergfeld MA, et al: Isolated skeletal involvement in Cushing's syndrome: response to therapy. J Clin Endocrinol Metab 52:1033–1038, 1982

26. Fachine JD, Zafar MS, Mellinger RC, et al: Pituitary carcinoma mimics the ectopic adrenocorticotropin syndrome. J Clin Endocrinol Metab 50:1062–1065, 1980

27. Lee PA, Weldon VV, Migeon CJ: Short stature as the only clinical sign of Cushing's syndrome. J Pediatr 86:8991, 1975

28. Saad MF, Adams F, Mackay B, et al: Occult Cushing's disease presenting with acute psychosis. Am J Med 76:759–766, 1984

29. Reus VI, Miner C: Evidence for physiological effects of hypercortisolemia in psychiatric patients. Psychiatry Res 14:47–56, 1985

30. Chrousos GP, Vingerhoeds A, Brandon D, et al: Primary cortisol resistance in man: a glucocorticoid receptor-mediated disease. J Clin Invest 69:1261–1269, 1982

31. Chrousos GP, Vingerhoeds ACM, Loriaux DL, et al: Primary cortisol resistance: a family study. J Clin Endocrinol Metab 56:1243–1245, 1983

32. Rubinow DR, Post RM, Gold PW, et al: The relationship between cortisol and clinical phenomenology of affective illness, in Neurobiology of Mood Disorders. Edited by Post RM, Ballenger JC. Baltimore, Williams & Wilkins, 1983

33. Fava GA, Carson SW, Perini GI: the metyrapone test in affective disorders and schizophrenia. J Affective Disord 6:241–247, 1984

34. Reus VI, Joseph M, Dallman M: Regulation of ACTH and cortisol in depression. Peptides 4:785–788, 1983

35. Carr D, Wool C, Lydiard R, et al: Rate sensitive inhibition of ACTH release in depression. Am J Psychiatry 141:590–592, 1984

36. Butler P, Besser G: Pituitary-adrenal function in severe depressive illness. Lancet 1:1234–1236, 1968

37. Winokur A, Amsterdam J, Caroff S, et al: Variability of hormonal responses to a series of neuroendocrine challenges in depressed patients. Am J Psychiatry 139:39–44, 1982

38. Carroll BJ: Control of plasma cortisol levels in depression: studies with the dexamethasone suppression test, in Depressive Illness: Some Research Studies. Edited by Davies B, Carroll BJ, Mowbray RM. Springfield, Ill, Charles C Thomas, 1972

39. Gold P, Chrousos G, Kellner C, et al: Psychiatric implications of basic and clinical studies with corticotropin releasing factor. Am J Psychiatry 141:619–627, 1984

40. Glass AR, Zavadil III AP, Halberg F, et al: Circadian rhythm of serum cortisol in Cushing's disease. J Clin Endocrinol Metab 59:161–165, 1984

41. Jordan RM, Ramos-Gabatin A, Kendall JW, et al: Dynamics of adrenocorticotropin (ACTH) secretion in cyclic Cushing's syndrome: evidence for more than one abnormal ACTH biorhythm. J Clin Endocrinol Metab 55:531–537, 1982

42. Liberman B, Wajchenberg BL, Tambascia MA, et al: Periodic remission in Cushing's disease with paradoxical dexamethasone response: an expression of periodic hormonogenesis. J Clin Endocrinol Metab 43:913–918, 1976

43. Brown RD, Van Loon GR, Orth DN, et al: Cushing's disease with periodic hormonogenesis: one explanation for paradoxical response to dexamethasone. J Clin Endocrinol Metab 36:445–451, 1973

44. Pasqualini RQ, Gurevich N: Spontaneous remission in a case of Cushing's syndrome. Journal of Clinical Endocrinology 16:406–411, 1956

45. Reed K, Watkins M, Dobson H: Mania in Cushing's syndrome: case report. J Clin Psychiatry 44:460–462, 1983

46. Becker L, Gold P, Chrousos G: Analogies between Cushing's disease and depression: a case report. Gen Hosp Psychiatry 5:89–91, 1983

47. Smith DJ, Kohler PC, Helminiak R: Intermittent Cushing's syndrome with an empty sella turcica. Arch Intern Med 142:2185–2187, 1982

48. Wolff SM, Adler RC, Buskirk ER, et al: A syndrome of periodic hypothalamic discharge. Am J Med 36:956–967, 1964

49. Zondek H, Leszynsky HE: Transient Cushing syndrome. Br Med J 16:197–200, 1956

50. Burch W: A survey of results with transsphenoidal surgery in Cushing's disease. N Engl J Med 308:103–104, 1983

51. Krieger DT: Physiopathology of Cushing's syndrome. Endocr Rev 4:22–43, 1983

52. Burrow G, Wortzman G, Newcastle N, et al: Microadenomas of the pituitary and abnormal cella tomograms in an unselected autopsy series. N Engl J Med 304:156–158, 1981

53. Laignel-Lavastine M, Jonnesco V: L'hypophyse des psychopathes. Encephale 1:25–45, 1913

54. Hsu T, Gann DS, Tsan K, et al: Cyproheptadine in the control of Cushing's disease. Johns Hopkins Medical Journal 149:77–83, 1981

55. Lankford HV, Tucker H. Blackard WG: A cyproheptadine-reversible defect in ACTH control persisting after removal of the pituitary tumor in Cushing's disease. N Engl J Med 305:1244–1248, 1981

56. Elias AN, Gwinup G, Balenta LJ: Effects of valproic acid, nalaxone and hydrocortisone in Nelson's syndrome and Cushing's disease. Journal of Clinical Endocrinology 15:151–154, 1981

57. Cavagnini F, Invitti C, Polli EE: Sodium valproate in Cushing's disease. Lancet 2:162–163, 1984

58. Price J, Ward G: Cyproheptadine in bipolar affective illness with Cushingoid features. Aus NZ J Psychiatry 11:201–202, 1977

59. Gold PW, Extein I, Ballenger JC, et al: Rapid mood cycling and concomitant cortisol changes produced by cyproheptadine. Am J Psychiatry 137:378–379, 1980

60. Kontula K, Mustajoki P, Paetau A, et al: Development of Cushing's disease in a patient with anorexia nervosa. J Endocrinol Invest 7:35–40, 1984

61. Fink M: Neuroendocrinology and ECT: a review of recent developments. Compr Psychiatry 21:450–459, 1980

62. Reis R, Bokau J: Electroconvulsive therapy following pituitary surgery. J Nerv Ment Dis 167:767–768, 1979

63. Albala A, Greden J, Tarika J, et al: Changes in serial dexamethasone suppression tests among unipolar depressives receiving ECT. Biol Psychiatry 16:551–560, 1981

64. Falk WE, Mahnke MW, Poskanzer DC: Lithium prophylaxis of corticotropin-induced psychosis. JAMA 241:1011–1012, 1979

65. Goggans FC, Weisberg LJ, Koran LM: Lithium prophylaxis of prednisone psychosis: a case report. J Clin Psychiatry 44:111–112, 1983

66. Smigan L, Perris C: Cortisol changes in long-term lithium therapy. Neuropsychobiology 11:219–223, 1984

Chapter 6

Depression in Drug Addicts and Alcoholics

Irl Extein, M.D.
Charles A. Dackis, M.D.
Mark S. Gold, M.D.
A. L. C. Pottash, M.D.

Chapter 6

Depression in Drug Addicts and Alcoholics

T he common coincidence of drug and alcohol dependence and depression raises complex possibilities for diagnosis and treatment. As alcohol and drug use becomes increasingly prevalent and increasingly recognized in patients seeking psychiatric care, it becomes more important for us to understand the nature of the interactions between drug and alcohol use and mood. Despite efforts by professionals to delineate clear-cut clinical syndromes, the psychiatric practitioner is becoming increasingly aware that a large percentage of patients come to psychiatric attention with a mix of psychiatric symptomatology and drug and alcohol abuse. This is particularly true among adolescents, where pure mood symptoms or pure substance abuse without changes in mood are rare. The reported prevalence of significant depressive symptoms ranged from about 30 to 60 percent in substance abusers admitted to treatment facilities (1–8). This chapter will focus attention on three of the most commonly used and serious addicting substances: opioids (primarily heroin and methadone), alcohol, and cocaine.

The biopsychosocial model of psychiatry suggests multiple mechanisms whereby drug and alcohol abuse affect mood and whereby changes in mood, particularly depression, lead to drug and alcohol abuse. First, consider the biological, psychological, and social aspects of chemical dependence that can affect mood. Data have accumulated suggesting that many individuals afflicted with drug and alcohol dependence are genetically predisposed. The strong influence of genetics in inheritance of alcoholism has been well documented, particularly by Scandinavian studies of adoptees (9). Certainly the biological influence of the drugs and alcohol themselves can affect central nervous system functioning and this represents another biological cause of mood changes in drug addicts and alcoholics. The psychological consequences of drug and alcohol abuse and dependence can also account for depressed mood, with loss of self-esteem, lack of productivity, and a loss of previous reinforcers. Likewise, the social consequences of drug and alcohol abuse include massive disruptions in family, friendship, and occupational ties that can account for significant depressed mood. The long-term physiological and psychosocial disruptions of drug abuse can lead to a final common pathway of depressed mood.

As clear as it is that chronic drug use and its physiological and psychosocial consequences can lead to depression, similarly psychiatric disturbances can predispose to drug and alcohol dependence. Patients prone to biological depression, including unipolar depressive illness and manic-depressive illness, may sometimes self-medicate. Some investigators have suggested that certain alcoholics and drug addicts should be listed as "secondary addicts" because of their tendency to abuse substances only when in the throes of a primary psychiatric episode such as a depression or mania. Clearly this is a minority of cases, but certainly a significant and treatable minority. Similarly, psychological and social problems and stress can predispose to drug abuse. There has been much debate in the literature over whether there exists an "addictive personality" (10). This has probably been overdone and is an oversimplified notion, yet certain personality traits, including immaturity, dependency, and antisocial traits, may be involved as predisposing factors to addiction. Social disruption, peer influence, and general societal and cultural trends also may predispose to certain kinds of drug and alcohol use. The fact that cocaine use is fashionable in some circles in American society in the 1980s is a factor that has caused many people to become involved in cocaine use.

Consider the main overall theories of the relationship of drug and alcohol dependence and depression. One possibility is that patients are simply self-medicating primary depressions. The second theory is that some patients have developed depressions as a physiological or psychosocial consequence of their addiction. The third is that patients who present with both depression and alcohol or drug dependence may simply have two illnesses.

This latter possibility of two coexisting illnesses should certainly be kept in mind. Psychiatrists, as other medical practitioners, should strive to think in terms of simple, singular explanations. But it should also be recognized that often patients have more than one common illness. Just as many patients have coronary artery disease and arthritis, or diabetes mellitus and manic-depressive illness, so many patients may have alcoholism or drug dependence and depressive illness. A recent major epidemiologic study (11) of disorders in the general population as defined by the *Diagnostic and Statistical Manual of*

Mental Disorders, Third Edition (DSM-III) (12) reported the following ranges of lifetime prevalence rates: alcohol abuse–dependence, 11.5 to 15.7 percent; drug abuse–dependence, 5.5 to 5.8 percent; major depression, 3.7 to 6.7 percent; and mania, 0.6 to 1.1 percent. Thus, based simply on random association, one would expect about 6 percent of alcoholics and drug addicts to have a major mood disorder.

With psychiatrists using the more sophisticated nosology of the Research Diagnostic Criteria (RDC) (13) and the DSM-III, they are becoming increasingly sophisticated about subtypes of depression. This is very important when considering the relationship between depression and drug and alcohol abuse. Not all depression represents primary major depressive illness. Many addicts may have mixed affective syndromes with significant depressive symptomatology but not clear enough to make criteria for major depression. Many addicts may have depressive symptomatology that waxes and wanes in relation to their substance use and their treatment. Addicts interviewed and assessed at different times over the course of their illness may meet criteria for different affective syndromes. For example, at one time a patient may meet criteria for dysthymic disorder, another time criteria for major depression, and yet at another time, perhaps during a condition of intoxication or withdrawal, criteria for an organic affective illness (12). Many of the depressive syndromes and symptom complexes seen during the early stages of inpatient treatment may represent, in fact, organic depressive syndromes. Some examples include intoxication and withdrawal states and mental status changes associated with medical problems such as infection. The practitioner would well heed the admonition of DSM-III that a psychiatric diagnosis is not to be given to a patient when there is a medical or neurological explanation for the symptoms.

Addicting substances are powerful mood-altering substances. Opioids, alcohol, and cocaine are powerful euphoric agents. In individuals predisposed to addiction, the reinforcing properties of the addictive substance can become more important to the individual than any other aspect of life, including sex, food, maintenance of health, and family, social, and occupational ties. Keeping this in mind, it is not surprising that patients with mood problems become involved in using drugs that affect mood. Likewise, it is not surprising that substances that affect mood and the biological central nervous system substrate of mood do cause temporary and sometimes permanent alterations in the biological mood-regulating systems that cause psychiatric symptomatology. This is an important general point to keep in mind. Many times addicts feel that because the high is temporary, the use of drugs and alcohol causes only temporary changes. This is not true. The drugs under discussion in this chapter interact with brain systems such as norepinephrine and endorphin systems that regulate normal mood functioning. Hence, chronic alterations of these by drugs such as cocaine, opioids, and alcohol can cause long-lasting changes in these chemical mood-regulating systems, and hence sometimes chronic alternatives in mood and other psychopathology.

Given the complexities of the relationship between alcohol and drugs and mood, it is doubly important to do a very careful diagnostic assessment of an individual who is addicted and has significant depressive symptomatology. This will be outlined in somewhat more detail below and also detailed under individual substances. The drug-free evaluation and reevaluation of the individual patient after detoxification is absolutely essential to the proper assessment of mood disturbance in an addicted individual and essential for formulating and carrying out a successful treatment plan.

Not only do the complex interactions between mood and addiction raise interesting academic questions, but these interactions are crucial to formulating and carrying out treatment. There have been many controversies in the area of treatment of addicts that have involved different treatment philosophies based on different understandings of the interactions between mood and addiction (14). This issue will be discussed in more detail later. It should be highlighted that there have been two poles of treatment approaches, although contemporary approaches are becoming much more sophisticated about integrating these poles. One pole has been the stereotypic "psychiatric" approach, aiming to do psychotherapy to find out why an individual drinks or uses drugs (while sometimes prescribing potentially addictive sedatives) without focusing in a pragmatic way on stopping the addiction and the systems that support the addiction. The other stereotype has been the stereotypic view of Alcoholics Anonymous (AA) (15), advocating cessation of drug and alcohol use with peer support without attention to concomitant psychiatric problems or need for psychiatric treatment. Much of the conflict between these two stereotypic extremes has been played out in the area of whether nonaddicting psychotropic drugs (such as lithium and tricyclic antidepressants) are appropriate for treating the proportion of addicts who may have significant psychiatric pathology even after detoxification.

We feel it is very important to state in the beginning that treatment should be interactive and should utilize modalities that benefit each individual patient. Certainly sophisticated medical and psychiatric evaluation and treatment are necessary and in some cases use of nonaddicting psychotropics can be essential for maintaining an individual's drug-free state and sobriety. We also feel that strong educational programs as well as peer support groups emphasizing ongoing recovery and total abstinence such as provided by AA and Narcotics Anonymous (NA) are essential. All of the above ingredients are best integrated in a hospital program in a structured therapeutic milieu.

POSTDETOXIFICATION DRUG-FREE NEUROPSYCHIATRIC EVALUATION

If there is one aspect of care of the drug addict or alcoholic that can cut across much of the complexity and confusion of the interaction between addiction and depression, it is the careful attention to a drug-free evaluation after the detoxification period. Clinicians and even patients and their families can get bogged down in unanswerable diagnostic and treatment dilemmas if the entire treatment plan is formulated and carried out when the individual is still under the strong physiological influence of recent drug use, and is still experiencing withdrawal symptoms.

Clearly, all drugs of abuse affect mood. Withdrawal states affect mood strongly. Neurovegetative symptoms such as disturbances in sleep, appetite, sexual function, and energy are often profoundly affected by the physiological effects of drugs and drug withdrawal. Cocaine is an excellent example of a drug whose intoxication and withdrawal states have profound effects on mood (16).

Cocaine intoxication causes a motoric hyperactivity and euphoric mood that clearly makes assessment of baseline functioning impossible. Likewise, the withdrawal state from cocaine, although controversial, probably includes some lowering of mood and energy that, again, makes assessment of mood very difficult.

We emphasize to our patients that an initial assessment is necessary to identify medical problems or a need for any acute psychiatric care, as well as to establish a working alliance with the patient and family. However, we also emphasize that we are more interested in knowing what an individual is like after detoxification than we are in knowing what he or she is like when either intoxicated or in withdrawal. These latter two states are only temporary and do not necessarily give important clues to long-range treatment needs.

Thus mood itself must be reassessed after detoxification. This length of time will vary from substance to substance. As a general rule of thumb, one must usually allow several weeks after drug use (be it street drug or drug used in the hospital for detoxification) in order to be able to get any realistic notion of what an individual is like.

Many patients have been addicted to drugs for years and they (and their families) have lost any realistic notion themselves of what their mood is like and what their personality structure is like in the drug-free state. Thus diagnostic interviews that aim to make the DSM-III diagnosis must often be re-done after the detoxification. Likewise, biological diagnostic tests such as the dexamethasone suppression test (DST) must be done at a reasonable time period after detoxification to avoid artifacts.

Many alcoholics and drug addicts may have been treated inappropriately with psychotropic medications based on symptomatology during the acute withdrawal stage of their illness (14). It is well known in treatment of depression in nonaddicts that there is a very high rate of placebo response and spontaneous recovery in depressive syndromes. This is probably even more true for addicts where there are so many complicating factors that could affect mood. Thus the results of antidepressant treatment during withdrawal are virtually impossible to interpret. This does not mean that patients who have significant mood and other psychiatric symptomatology *after* detoxification should not be appropriately treated with psychotropics.

It is our finding, which will be outlined in detail further on, that the rate of major depressive illness postdetoxification is much higher in opioid addicts (particularly methadone addicts) and in cocaine addicts than it is in alcoholics (7, 8, 14). The reasons for this are not entirely clear, but may reflect long-term physiological adaptive changes in endorphin, dopamine, and norepinephrine systems that affect mood even weeks after detoxification has been completed. The initial evaluation and postdetoxification period reevaluation also allow for assessment and treatment of the multiple medical problems (17) that can compound addiction. For example, nutritional deficiencies including covert and overt vitamin deficiencies, intercurrent infection, and chronic disease can certainly affect mood. It is important to see how the mood changes with good medical care and nutrition.

It is our experience that many treatment dilemmas and affectively charged differences in treatment philosophies among different staff members become much less intense and often disappear if one gives careful attention to a drug-free evaluation. It is difficult to disagree with prescription of psychotropic medication (e.g., tricyclic antidepressants) in an individual who, 4 weeks after entry into an alcoholism program and 2 weeks after completion of detoxification meets criteria for major depression. Likewise, it is difficult to lobby for psychotropic medication or need for intensive insight-oriented psychotherapy in a patient who met criteria for major depression on entry into a treatment program, but 2 weeks after completion of detoxification is showing a positive mood change and positive involvement in a recovery program.

As in most other aspects of medicine, the dictum in treating mood disturbance in addicts is not to treat until the physician is sure what is being treated, and then to treat it appropriately and aggressively. The prescription of addicting psychotropic medications such as barbiturate or benzodiazepine sedatives in the alcoholic not only can perpetuate the addiction (and give physicians a bad name), but can also interfere with the necessary first step of drug-free evaluation.

A number of medical aspects (17) of alcoholism and drug abuse that can affect mood should be mentioned. Vitamin deficiencies (e.g., B1, B6, B12, and folic acid) were mentioned above. In addition, infections that are common in intravenous drug addicts, such as viral hepatitis and subacute bacterial endocarditis, can affect mood. Endocarditis can result in embolic phenomena to the brain that can affect mood as well as general intellectual functioning. Drug and alcohol abuse—via the mechanisms of toxic effects, related medical illnesses, or seizures or head injuries related to drug or alcohol use—can cause organic brain damage with change in mood, including depression, just as can occur in organic brain syndromes from other causes.

OPIOID ADDICTION (HEROIN AND METHADONE)

Opium derivatives and their contemporary synthetic relatives are among the most powerful euphoriants known. Many pharmacological agents have been used to effect detoxification from these substances, which are strongly physiologically addicting (18). In the modern psychopharmacological era, methadone, which is orally active and long acting, has been used both for detoxification and for psychosocial stabilization. Methadone certainly had its advantages in helping to socialize patients by taking them off the streets and away from the criminal activities often utilized to obtain money to buy heroin. However, methadone maintenance itself has had some drawbacks, including continued maintenance on an addictive drug with attendant physiological consequences, and difficulty detoxifying from methadone itself. More recently, clonidine has emerged as the treatment of choice for opioid withdrawal and represents the technology for detoxifying many addicts who heretofore might have had to stay on methadone maintenance (19). Whatever the pharmacological issues in detoxification, it has become appreciated that the continuation of a drug-free state following any detoxification is the most challenging and problematic goal for the opioid addict, the medical community, and society. In general, rehabilitation results have not been very good.

One focus of study of the opioid addict has been the relationship between mood changes and addiction. Although basically a central nervous system depressant, opioids are mood elevators in the sense that they cause a euphoric state of perceived well-being. It would be natural to think that depressed mood predisposes to opioid addiction and opioid use might cause long-standing mood changes. Studies of acute versus chronic administration of heroin found that although acute administration produced euphoria, chronic administration produced increased hostility, agitation, and depression (20).

Many studies of depression in opioid addicts have measured only severity of depression without regard to RDC or DSM-III diagnostic criteria. A major study of depression in opiate addicts was performed by Rounsaville et al. (5) at Yale. They did a very sophisticated diagnostic and clinical assessment of methadone maintenance patients. Depressive symptomatology was found in a significant proportion of the methadone maintenance addicts. Rounsaville et al. (1) found that 17 percent of opioid addicts entering a multi-modality drug treatment program met RDC for current major depression. Kleber and Gold (2) found that 30 percent of patients in a methadone treatment program met DSM-III criteria for major depression. Rounsaville and Kleber (21) have reported an interesting lack of diagnostic reliability over time in the assessment of depression in opioid addicts. Mirin et al. (6) found that among opioid addicts admitted to inpatient treatment, 18 percent meet DSM-III criteria for major (unipolar) depression and 3 percent for bipolar depression.

However, with the ability to detoxify patients using clonidine and other future, better methods, the issue of mood disturbance in detoxified addicts may be even more important. The area is complex. It may be that syndromes in opioid addicts either before or after detoxification that meet DSM-III criteria for major depression may be clinically distinct from depressive syndromes that appear similar that occur in the nonaddictive population.

Similarity of depressive symptoms in addicts and nonaddicts does not necessarily imply common etiology, common course, or common responses to treatment. Rounsaville et al. (1) found that 17 percent of their patients satisfied RDC for current major depression, and that there was a 48 percent lifetime prevalence of RDC major depression in the methadone addicts. Of note was that 95 percent of those with the lifetime diagnosis of major depression experienced their first depressive episode only after the onset of opioid abuse. Certainly this finding does not support the notion that the methadone addicts were using heroin or other opiates initially to self-medicate preexisting depression. It is difficult to see someone in the throes of a major depression with all the attendant apathy and dysfunction developing the wherewithal to pay for and obtain heroin.

Our treatment facilities have focused on detoxification of opioid-dependent patients and intensive inpatient and then outpatient treatment with the aim of abstinence from all drugs of abuse. Appropriate psychiatric treatment, including psychotropic medications when indicated, as well as a therapeutic milieu, family involvement, and support groups are utilized.

We have reported on a series of 80 detoxified opioid addicts, 21 dependent on methadone and 59 dependent on heroin (7). All the methadone-dependent patients were detoxified with clonidine, whereas 31 of the heroin patients were detoxified with minimal amounts of methadone as needed for periods of several days. The remaining heroin-dependent patients required detoxification with clonidine after stabilization on methadone. This study excluded patients with active hepatitis. It should be noted that the methadone-dependent patients experienced more abstinence symptoms and required higher doses of clonidine for longer periods of time than the heroin-dependent patients.

The Schedule for Affective Disorders and Schizophrenia Current Status (SADS-C) (22) was used as an interview tool for diagnosis. This SADS-C interview was conducted 2 to 3 weeks after detoxification so as to be able to avoid merely assessing the effects of the methadone, the clonidine, or the withdrawal state. After detoxification, 13 (62 percent) of the methadone-addicted patients and 15 (25 percent) of the heroin-addicted patients met RDC for major depressive illness.

Thus the increased prevalence of major depression in methadone addicts parallels the more prolonged and symptomatic detoxification in the methadone addicts. Perhaps the methadone, being a long-acting, potent opioid readily available to clinic patients, caused a more profound disruption of central nervous system function than did heroin. Heroin has a shorter half-life and is more expensive on the street than methadone in clinics, and may cause less complete disruption of naturally occurring endogenous opioid (endorphin) systems.

The greater prevalence of major depression in methadone patients compared to heroin addicts could reflect an organic affective syndrome resulting from protracted withdrawal or persistent disruption in brain mechanisms by methadone (7). Certainly the so-called chronic abstinence syndrome of the methadone addicts is well documented.

Even after the acute withdrawal symptoms that usually last about 2 weeks subside, patients have a number of chronic symptoms including low energy, anhedonia, irritability, and insomnia. The insomnia is reasonably objective and noted not infrequently for sometimes months at a time after detoxification from methadone. These symptoms are even more prevalent in patients who have been on high-dose methadone (greater than 30 mg a day of methadone) from a clinic for many years at a time. Even sensitivities of respiratory drive to carbon dioxide suppression have been shown to be abnormal for months at a time in opioid addicts after detoxification. Thus there is a true protracted abstinence syndrome (23) after detoxification from opioids, which may cause a protracted organic syndrome that includes depression. We will report later on data on use of neuroendocrine diagnostic tests, such as the DST, to establish biological markers for true major depressive illness in the detoxified opioid addict.

The higher rate of major depression in our study compared to that of Rounsaville et al. (1) may reflect the fact that the patients in our study had been detoxified. There may be rebound depression occurring after the cessation of opioids. A depression occurring for whatever reason after detoxification could motivate the patient to self-medicate with opioids at the very time of greatest vulnerability to relapse, and may explain the high rates of relapse in detoxified opioid addicts. Certainly anecdotally, many patients crave opioids not just for the euphoric effect but in an effort to relieve their chronic withdrawal symptomatology.

In general, reports of tricyclic antidepressant treatment of methadone maintenance patients with significant depressive symptomatology have not been very positive (7). This may reflect simply the fact that the kind of depression common in methadone addicts is different from the usual major depression in nonaddicts and not amenable to tricyclic treatment. Alternatively, this essentially poor therapeutic performance may simply reflect that depression in methadone addicts is heterogeneous and the subgroup of true major depressions within this group of dysphoric addicts might indeed respond to tricyclics. There has been little research on the psychopharmacological treatment of depression in detoxified opioid addicts, probably because of the difficulties with detoxification and recidivism.

It has been our finding, which will be discussed in more detail later, that tricyclics, as well as other psychotropic medications including lithium and monoamine oxidase inhibitors (MAOI), can be important adjuncts to postdetoxification inpatient treatment and the outpatient recovery phase of treatment in opioid addicts. We have, in fact, found that in opioid addicts, treatment with antidepressant medication is associated with a higher likelihood of avoidance of relapse to opioid use, independent of attendance in outpatient follow-up (24).

It is interesting to speculate on the physiological substrate in the brain of the relatively high rate of depression in detoxified methadone addicts. The discovery in the early 1970s of naturally occurring opioid receptors in the brain led shortly thereafter to the discovery of naturally occurring opioid peptides in the brain (endorphins and enkephalins) (25). There are neurons in the brain that utilize endorphins and enkephalins as neuromodulators or neurotransmitters. It has been suggested that these neurological systems are involved in regulating such functions as pain perception, response to stress, and mood. Effects of opioids in depression have been studied, and abnormal neuroendocrine responses to opioids in depression have been reported (26, 27).

Opioid addiction would be expected to cause opioid receptor down-regulation and feedback inhibition of production of naturally occurring neuronal endorphins and enkephalins (see Figure 1). The latter would be analogous to the shutting down of adrenal production of corticosteroids in patients who are treated with high doses of corticosteroids on a protracted basis. Simply put, the homeostatic mechanisms of the brain of a methadone addict would "see" that

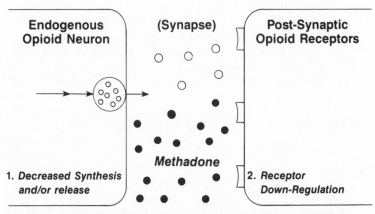

Figure 1. A possible mechanism for depression following detoxification from addiction to methadone or other opioids. Proposed post-synaptic opioid receptor down-regulation and feedback inhibition of presynaptic endogenous opioid synthesis or release secondary to chronic addiction to methadone or other opioids.

there was no need for the endorphins and enkephalins and these would no longer be produced. Following detoxification, there may be a long delay before the brain and neuroendocrine systems begin again to make the naturally occurring opioid peptides. Thus after detoxification there may be a relative endorphin and enkephalin deficiency state that could account for some of the depressive picture seen clinically.

We have reported data on the decreased adrenocorticotropic hormone (ACTH) response to naloxone in methadone compared to heroin addicts, suggesting that endorphin systems are deficient in methadone addicts as opposed to heroin addicts after detoxification (28). This presents an interesting therapeutic paradox involving methadone maintenance. Although methadone maintenance may have advantages in socialization of street heroin addicts, there may be long-term disadvantages in that the individual is more thoroughly addicted and may have a more difficult time returning to drug-free living. This notion is also supported by the finding of a blunted cortisol response to ACTH in chronic methadone addicts (29). This is a pattern consistent with chronically low ACTH and therefore low endorphin levels. The interaction of endogenous opioid peptide systems and norepinephrine systems must also be considered (19). Endogenous opioid peptides exert a tonic inhibition on norepinephrine neurons in the locus ceruleus, which is thought to be involved in depression.

Several studies have addressed the use of antidepressants in opioid addicts. Spensley (30) treated 27 methadone addicts with doxepin in an uncontrolled study and found that 25 reported improvement. Woody et al. (31) conducted a double-blind study with doxepin in 35 depressed methadone addicts and found significant improvement in depression and decrease in craving for heroin. Kleber et al. (32) studied 46 methadone-maintained addicts and found improvement in depression with both the imipramine- and placebo-treated groups. These two groups did not differ significantly with respect to improvement and Kleber et al. concluded that most depression in addicts would remit spontaneously. Given the extremely high rate of relapse to drug use of the opioid addicts following detoxification and treatment, and given the lethality of opioid addiction, we consider it important to utilize pharmacotherapy along with any other means of productive treatment for each individual case. Our follow-up studies of a population of patients which included many opioid addicts have suggested that antidepressants have an independent efficacy in a recovery program (24).

Woody et al. (33) reported the results of a study on the effects of psychotherapy on the functioning of heroin addicts who were on methadone maintenance at the time of the study. The patients had been on methadone for less than 6 months. Both cognitive-behavioral psychotherapy and supportive-expressive psychotherapy, in contrast to paraprofessional drug counseling alone, improved functioning in patients with more severe psychiatric symptoms. This psychotherapy effect was not noted in patients whose psychiatric symptoms were of a low severity.

ALCOHOLISM

Alcoholism represents the most common addiction in the United States, with lifetime prevalence of alcohol dependence or abuse reportedly up to 15 percent (11). Much of what will be said about alcoholism could be applied to addiction to sedative medication (such as benzodiazepines and barbiturates).

The AA treatment philosophy has become a critical part of addiction treatment programs. AA sees alcoholism as a life-long disease over which the patient is powerless as an individual. Sobriety requires participation in the larger peer group of recovery groups (14, 15).

Alcohol can affect thinking and behavior as well as mood on a physical basis. Alcohol intoxication and withdrawal syndromes are well documented (13, 34). Alcohol intoxication is associated with depressed mood, behavioral disinhibition, and amnesia. Withdrawal is associated with anxiety, delirium, and hallucinosis.

There is a whole gamut of physical systems failures that can be caused by alcohol. The most common forms of specific organ damage seen in alcoholics are cirrhosis of the liver, peripheral neuropathy, brain damage, cardiomyopathy, gastritis, pancreatitis, and anemia. Inadequate nutrition may play a role in alcohol's toxic effects on the liver and the nervous system (17). The effects of a major system dysfunction such as hepatic dysfunction from alcoholic hepatitis or cirrhosis can certainly affect mood on a physiological basis.

As mentioned in the introduction, there has been much confusion and controversy over the relationships between depressed mood and alcoholism (4, 14, 34), much of it resulting from confusion and lack of consistency as to the point in the course of the illness and its treatment at which mood is assessed. The concept of primary and secondary psychiatric illness (13, 35) can help clarify the relationships between alcoholism and depressed mood. Certainly secondary depressions in alcoholics (i.e., depression following addiction and related to addiction or withdrawal) are more common than primary depressions (unipolar or bipolar), which occur in a significant proportion of alcoholics and require psychopharmacological treatment

(4, 7, 14, 34). A recent study of primary diagnostic groups among alcoholics has shown the primary affective disorder group to be a small but significant subgroup (34). Data suggest that genetic factors play a major role in the development of primary alcoholism (9, 35). The notion of "secondary alcoholism" has also emerged to describe patients who drink only when in a depressive or manic episode.

Our group has studied 70 consecutive patients admitted to our alcoholism rehabilitation programs and assessed diagnostically for depression (7). The SADS-C interviews were done on patients who filled RDC for alcohol dependence and were interviewed 2 to 3 weeks after the completion of alcohol detoxification with chlordiazepoxide. Although a large number of these patients appeared quite depressed on admission, only 5 (7 percent) of 70 met RDC for major depression in postdetoxified opioid addicts. These data are certainly against the self-medication theory of alcoholism. If individuals with primary depressive illness were commonly self-medicating, one might expect more self-medication of depression with the legal and easily obtainable alcohol than with heroin or methadone and hence a higher rate of postdetoxification depression in alcoholics compared to opioid addicts. In fact, the contrary was found true. These data again suggest that there may be something specific to the postmethadone detoxification state that contributes to depression.

COCAINE ABUSE AND ADDICTION

There is an epidemic of cocaine abuse currently in the United States, particularly in middle and upper income groups and in the higher educational and occupational strata of society (36, 37). Cocaine is a short-acting euphoric agent that causes hyperactive euphoric states (16, 38). Cocaine's effects depend in some degree on the route of administration of the drug, with increasingly potent effects from intranasal use (snorting), inhalation (free-basing), and intravenous use. The intense high usually lasts less than half an hour and is followed by an intense "crash" with marked depressed symptomatology. There is still some dispute as to whether cocaine is truly addicting. However, if one defines addiction in terms of compulsive drug-seeking behavior with severe negative consequences, then cocaine is a highly addicting drug (16, 36, 37). Cocaine addicts have been reported to have a rate of major depression as high as 50 percent.

We studied 34 (28 men) consecutive patients in whom cocaine was the primary drug of abuse and who were admitted to a private psychiatric hospital for evaluation and treatment (8). This sample represented a primarily middle to upper class group of suburban addicts; 28 were white and 27 were employed, with a mean age of

29 years. The patients were treated supportively for physiological and psychological symptoms of withdrawal. There does usually seem to be a mild physiological and psychological withdrawal state with low energy, depressed mood, insomnia, irritability, and cocaine craving.

The patients were assessed using semi-structured interviews of themselves and their family and applying DSM-III criteria at least 1 week following cessation of cocaine use. Of the 34 patients, 11 (32 percent) met DSM-III criteria for major depressive disorders (10 unipolar and 1 bipolar). Criteria for either atypical depression or dysthymic disorder was met by 16 patients who had significant depressive symptomatology but not of a nature, severity, or duration to meet criteria for major depression. Of interest is the fact that 4 of the patients met criteria for bipolar disorder (either manic or hypomanic) and 5 met criteria for attention deficit disorder. In addition, 18 had personality disorders: primarily borderline, antisocial, and narcissistic personalities. In addition, 26 abused other drugs, mostly alcohol or cannabis or both.

The relatively high prevalence of major depression in the cocaine abusers is consistent with previous reports. Mirin et al. (6) reported that 31 percent of newly admitted stimulant abusers met DSM-III criteria for major (unipolar) depression. The frequency of affective disorders (major depression most commonly) in the first-degree relatives of these stimulant abusers was 14 percent for males and 27 percent for females, 2 to 4 times higher than the frequencies of affective disorders in first-degree relatives of patients abusing opioids or depressants (6).

After being drug-free for 3 weeks, the stimulant abusers in the study of Mirin et al. (6) had significantly lower platelet monoamine oxidase levels than the other drug abuser groups. The stimulant abusers with retarded depressions also tended to have low or normal urinary excretion of 3-methoxy-4-hydroxyphenylglycol. These biological findings may reflect a biological vulnerability of cocaine and other stimulant abusers to depression, or else the biological consequences of stimulant abuse. These data as well as our own raise the question of whether a subgroup of cocaine abusers are self-medicating their depressions. It would be interesting to do further follow-up studies and examine whether depression pre-dated cocaine abuse or followed the beginning of cocaine abuse.

In a survey of 500 cocaine abusers randomly selected from more than 70,000 telephone callers to the 800-COCAINE Help Line, the callers' subjective reports of depression were assessed (37). Of these callers, 83 percent related significant depression as part of their cocaine use. In addition, 76 percent reported chronic fatigue and 82 percent reported sleep disturbance. Thus depressive symptomatology is common among cocaine users. In addition to the possibility that there is a subgroup of cocaine abusers who are self-medicating, another subgroup may have developed depression as a result of cocaine abuse (the so-called crash), possibly caused by down-regulation of brain norepinephrine systems.

One mechanism of action of cocaine that seems to be related to its euphoric effect is that cocaine potentiates catecholamine neuronal transmission in the central nervous system, particularly in dopaminergic pleasure centers in the brain (16, 39). Cocaine blocks the neuronal reuptake of dopamine and norepinephrine as well as causing direct release into the synapse of these neurotransmitters. These effects of cocaine have some mechanisms in common with both amphetamines and tricyclic antidepressants. One would expect this chronic facilitation of dopaminergic and noradrenergic neurotransmission possibly to lead to decreased presynaptic production of dopamine and norepinephrine. Data suggest that chronic cocaine use leads to a presynaptic dopamine deficiency state (39, 40) (Figure 2). The observed increased postsynaptic dopamine and norepinephrine receptor binding in animal studies of chronic cocaine use, as well as the reported increased serum prolactin in detoxifying cocaine addicts (41) are consistent with the dopamine deficiency hypothesis. Fol-

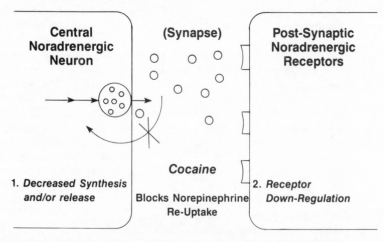

Figure 2. A possible mechanism for depression following cessation of chronic cocaine abuse. Proposed depletion of dopaminergic neuronal systems secondary to chronic cocaine abuse.

lowing cessation of cocaine use, brain dopamine or norepinephrine depletion may be the physiological substrate of the cocaine withdrawal syndrome, which includes prominent depression in addition to lack of energy and intense craving for cocaine (39, 40). A practical application of this theory has been the reported efficacy of the dopamine agonist bromocriptine in relieving the symptoms of cocaine withdrawal (42). The dopamine deficiency hypothesis of cocaine withdrawal would be analogous to the proposed deficit in endogenous opioid systems following detoxification from methadone.

It is our clinical experience that the majority of cocaine addicted patients go through a mildly to moderately intense low energy depression that is ameliorated by bromocriptine and remits spontaneously in several weeks with supportive care in a structured inpatient setting. Vitamin and amino acid (tyrosine) supplementation may be useful adjuncts (16) to a temporary use of low doses of nonaddicting psychotropic medications during this withdrawal phase. However, a significant minority of cocaine-addicted patients do not experience spontaneous remission of their low energy depression and go on to develop what appears to be a full-blown depressive syndrome. These depressions again are usually characterized by a lack of energy. Many such patients will respond positively to tricyclic antidepressant treatment, particularly the less sedating noradrenergic-type tricyclics such as nortriptyline or desipramine. In our study (8), 4 out of 5 patients with a major depression treated with tricyclic antidepressants of the noradrenergic type had good clinical responses. It seems sensible that the noradrenergic type antidepressant would be useful in cocaine abusers who may have depleted their noradrenergic systems. In our experience, these patients with postcocaine depression are exquisitely sensitive to the side effects of antidepressant medication, particularly sedation.

Several groups have investigated the efficacy of tricyclic antidepressants in maintaining abstinence in cocaine abusers. Reports of open studies suggest that use of imipramine or desipramine significantly decreases the craving and facilitates the detoxification of cocaine abusers (43, 44). This finding is still controversial and further studies utilizing placebo control and double-blind design, as well as strict monitoring for drug abuse in the follow-up period, need to be performed.

The subgroups of manic or hypomanic and attention deficit disorder patients among the cocaine addicts are very interesting. Mirin et al. (6) reported that 22 percent of newly admitted stimulant abusers met DSM-III criteria for bipolar disorder. This percentage of bipolar disorders was much higher than the 3 percent among opioid addicts and 6 percent among those addicted to depressants (e.g., diazepam, methaqualone).

It seems somewhat paradoxical that cocaine, which can cause manic and hypomanic symptoms, might be used by patients who have persistent hypomania or mania. These patients in our study were patients who had hypomania and mania that persisted after the detoxification period. It may be that as a manifestation of manic mood, patients seek to elevate that mood even further by using cocaine. It may also be that hypomanic or cyclothymic individuals, as part of their lifestyle, would be predisposed to use a so-called chic new drug such as cocaine. In our study (8) lithium was effective in the 4 patients with persistent manic or hypomanic symptoms. Neuroleptic medications were effectively used for patients with manic symptoms or poor impulse control.

The subgroup of patients with attention deficit disorder may well represent patients who were self-medicating themselves with the stimulant cocaine for their adult attention deficit disorder (13). Some of these patients may be effectively treated with desipramine and some may be effectively treated with medically controlled prescription of stimulants, such as methylphenidate. Given the addictive patterns of these patients, however, one would be rather reluctant to use addicting stimulants as a therapeutic regimen. Again, in the treatment of patients with cocaine abuse or addiction, as with the other types of addiction, the key to successful treatment is to defer major treatment decisions including use of psychotropics until at least a week or two after the patient's last drug use.

OTHER ADDICTING DRUGS

Although this chapter will not go into detailed discussion on the relationship of all drugs of abuse to depression, it should be noted that all abusable and addicting drugs affect mood acutely, from chronic use and from withdrawal. One common syndrome that should be noted is the so-called burn-out syndrome, common to a number of drugs including alcohol, marijuana, LSD, phencyclidine (PCP), and methadone. This syndrome includes chronic apathy, low energy, and inability to function in a meaningful way in society, usually with some intellectual deterioration. This seems to be a final common pathway of patients who abused any one of a number of addicting drugs on a chronic and long-term basis. This burn-out syndrome may well represent a form of subcortical and cortical brain damage that is only partially reversible. It may be seen as a depressive syndrome, probably an organic affective disorder, requiring careful neuropsychiatric assessment in each individual patient.

TREATMENT OUTCOME IN PATIENTS ADDICTED TO HEROIN, METHADONE, OR COCAINE

In an effort to assess factors associated with good and poor response to treatment, Ockert et al. (24) followed 101 patients at Fair Oaks Hospital in Summit, New Jersey, through inpatient treatment and up to 6 months of outpatient follow-up. This group of patients was a predominantly upper and middle class white suburban group of educated and employed addicts and thus somewhat different and unique compared to previous studies of outcome, which have focused on lower socioeconomic class addict populations with higher proportions of black addicts.

The average patient was a 29-year-old white Catholic male with 2 years of college education who earned $45,000 yearly and had been addicted for 7 years. Of the 101 patients, 25 were addicted to heroin, 22 to methadone, 19 to mixed opioids, 13 to cocaine, and 22 to "speedballs" (heroin combined with cocaine). Of these patients, 74 patients completed the inpatient program, which consisted of clonidine detoxification if needed, a psychiatric evaluation, and treatment including psychotropic medication if indicated. In addition, 51 patients entered the outpatient aftercare program, which emphasized group support and abstinence from drugs of abuse. Patients were rated using the Addiction Severity Index on admission and were rated again 6 months later.

At follow-up, 47 percent of the original patients were drug-free. The highest recidivism rate was in methadone addicts, followed by heroin addicts, speedball addicts, and cocaine abusers. Cocaine abusers were significantly more likely to be drug-free than opioid addicts. The following factors were associated with drug-free outcome: successful completion of the inpatient program, entry into the outpatient program, outpatient length of stay, presence of social support, and treatment with psychotropic medication (primarily tricyclic antidepressants).

The 25 patients treated with psychotropics were significantly ($p < .003$) more likely to be drug-free at follow-up (76 percent), independent of other variables, than were the 67 patients not given psychotropic medication (40 percent). These results suggest that subgroups of drug abusers benefit from appropriate use of psychotropic medication, possibly to treat depressive symptomatology or correct neurochemical deficits that may follow long-term drug use. Certainly the results of this study are not consistent with the fear that appropriate use of nonaddicting psychotropic medications interferes with the recovery phase of treatment.

NEUROENDOCRINE DIAGNOSTIC TESTS FOR MAJOR DEPRESSION IN DRUG ADDICTS AND ALCOHOLICS

Given the many confounding variables that can affect the diagnosis of depression in an addicted population, an objective marker for true biological depression would be extremely helpful. If found, such a marker would help the clinician to identify which of the depressed addicts were potential candidates for antidepressant medications.

In considering any laboratory diagnostic test, the possibility must be considered that drug and alcohol abuse can cause artifacts in the testing. For example, drug-induced and alcohol-induced changes in liver enzymes can cause changes in the rate of degradation of test substances, such as the dexamethasone used in the DST (45). The effect of alcohol on the hypothalamic-pituitary-adrenal (HPA) axis is dramatically seen in alcohol-induced pseudo-Cushing's syndrome (46). A number of studies in the literature on the DST as a diagnostic marker for depression in alcoholics have been confounded by failure to screen patients for hepatic dysfunction, alcohol withdrawal, and type of depressive symptomatology. Swartz and Dunner (47) reported a 33 percent incidence of DST nonsuppression in alcoholics who did not meet clinical criteria for the diagnosis of major depressive illness, suggesting that the specificity of the DST for major depression in alcoholics was very low.

In an effort to examine whether alcoholism itself caused artifactual nonsuppression on the DST, we studied the DST in a group of 20 nonalcoholics and 32 chronic alcoholics who were carefully screened to exclude major depression as well as hepatic disease (48). Patients fulfilling RDC on the SADS-C interview for major or minor depressive illness, hypomania, or mania were excluded from the study. Patients with bilirubin greater than 2.0 mg/100 ml albumin, less than 3.5 g/100 ml anemia, or present or past liver disease were also excluded from the study. This study aimed to discover whether alcoholism per se, independent of the hepatic effects and depression, would alter the 1-mg DST. Postdexamethasone cortisol levels were determined at 8:00 A.M., 4:00 P.M., and midnight. Cortisol level by radioimmunoassay greater than 5 μg/100 ml at any of the above time-points was considered nonsuppression. Of the 32 chronic alcoholics, 15 had a DST both during their initial week of alcohol withdrawal and following completion of the detoxification. During week 1, 3 of the 15 patients with alcohol withdrawal syndrome failed to suppress on the DST. After 3 weeks of sobriety, there were no DST abnormalities in the 32 chronic alcoholics.

The same patients were also administered a thyrotropin-releasing hormone (TRH) test as described in previous reports (49). The mean delta thyroid-stimulating hormone (TSH) during withdrawal of 7.3 μIU/ml was significantly lower than that of 9.6 μIU/ml after detoxification. Of the 15 patients with alcohol withdrawal at admission, 8 had a blunted TSH response to TRH when using the cut-off criterion of 7.0 μIU/ml and 5 had a blunted TSH response when using the more conservative and less sensitive criteria of 5.0 μIU/ml to define an abnormal TSH response. Of the 32 patients tested during week 4 after detoxification, 8 showed a TSH response of less than 7.0 μUI/ml.

More of the 15 patients tested during alcohol withdrawal than of the 20 nonalcoholics or the 32 alcoholics without alcohol withdrawal had DST and TRH test abnormalities. When performed after 3 weeks of sobriety, however, the DST but not the TRH test seemed to have potential as a specific laboratory adjunct in the diagnosis of depression in alcoholics. This is consistent with Loosen and Prange's (50) suggestion that a blunted TSH response to TRH is a trait marker for alcoholism. It clearly seems that the DST may have some potential as a diagnostic marker for depression in detoxified alcoholics, given the finding that alcohol dependence per se does not seem to cause DST nonsuppression. Further studies that include depressed and nondepressed alcoholics are needed. However, the TRH test is not a useful marker for major depression in an alcoholic population. It should be noted that the TRH test may still be extremely useful in identifying thyroid difficulties, especially early or subclinical hypothyroidism (51) in alcoholic patients.

Opioids have been reported to introduce artifacts in neuroendocrine testing. Certainly the interrelationship of beta endorphin and ACTH (52)—having a common precursor peptide—point out the relationship between changes in endogenous opioid systems and changes in the HPA axis. Opioid administration lowers cortiosol (53) and may cause blunting of the TSH response to TRH (54). Given the high rate of major depression in detoxified opioid addicts and the important theoretical and treatment question of whether this depression represents the same kind of depression as exists in non-addicts, it would be important to apply diagnostic markers such as the DST to the heroin and methadone addict population.

Dackis et al. (55) administered the DST as outlined above to 42 opioid addicts 2 weeks after detoxification. The patients included 27 heroin-dependent and 15 methadone-dependent patients. Within 3 days of the DST, each patient was administered a SADS-C by the same rater to determine whether the RDC for major depression were met. Patients were drug-free at the time of testing. This study reported that after detoxification, RDC major depression was present in 15 (36 percent) of the 42 opioid-dependent patients, including 9 (60 percent) of the 15 methadone-dependent patients and 6 (22 percent) of the 27 heroin-dependent patients. Of the 15 patients with RDC major depression, 12 failed to suppress on the DST. Only 2 of the 27 addicts without major depression failed to suppress.

The DST provided a sensitivity of 80 percent and a specificity of 93 percent for major depression in this population. These sensitivity and specificity figures are similar to those found for major depression using the DST as a marker in a nonaddict population. It is remarkable that, given the complexities of assessing depression in the postdetoxified opioid addict, the DST seems to be a sensitive and specific laboratory test for major depression in this population. It will certainly be important to follow up and find the relationships of both clinical diagnosis and laboratory markers to the clinical outcome, including long-term course and response to antidepressant medications. The possibility that methadone has some direct effects on both the HPA axis and on mood must be considered (28, 29).

There are fewer data on the effects of cocaine on neuroendocrine diagnostic tests than on the effects of alcohol and opioids. Data suggest that acute cocaine use causes blunting of the TSH response to TRH in a manner similar to the blunting caused by acute amphetamine intoxication. TRH testing of drug-free cocaine abusers (8) after detoxification showed 8 of 18 patients to have a blunted TSH response and 1 to have subclinical hypothyroidism. DST nonsuppression occurred with somewhat lower frequency in this population. Statistically significant relationships between DST and TRH test abnormalities and the diagnosis of major depression in the cocaine abusers were not noted.

TREATING DEPRESSION IN DRUG ADDICTS AND ALCOHOLICS

How one conceptualizes the relationship of depressed mood in an addict to the overall addictive process will determine much about treatment approach. We have outlined an individualized approach emphasizing the drug-free assessment of each patient following detoxification that would allow for the fact that there might be different factors operating in different patients, and hence need for individualization of treatment focus. Clearly, some aspects of treatment apply to almost all addicts, including evaluating, detoxification, the need to avoid return to use of all addicting substances (including alcohol), and the need to maintain involvement with structured inpatient and then outpatient follow-up programs utilizing AA or NA principles. The need for education about the nature of addictive illnesses for the individual and family is almost universal. The timing of all aspects of treatment would depend on the individual. For example, patients with severe depressive or other psychiatric syndromes would benefit more from the didactic and educational aspects as well as the peer support aspects of treatment after effective psychopharmacological treatment of the depression.

In our treatment programs, we have attempted to unite the principles of biological psychiatry and the principles of AA (14). We have found that these principles are reconcilable and mesh very well in a sophisticated treatment program utilizing a multidisciplinary treatment team. It is crucial, however, to maintain a good working relationship among staff members of different backgrounds, such as the psychiatrist who has no personal experience with addiction and the recovering addict counselor with a strong AA orientation.

Generally speaking, we have found that the vast majority of alcoholics do not require psychopharmacological or specific psychiatric intervention, although the majority of opioid addicts, cocaine abusers, and more complicated polydrug addicts do. We find that if psychiatry acknowledges some of the difficulties of purely psychiatric approaches to alcoholism and drug addiction, and if AA-oriented treatment acknowledges the ineffectiveness of purely AA approaches to someone suffering from an untreated major psychiatric syndrome, then there is much less friction between the two disciplines of psychiatry and AA or NA counseling.

We find two important items in integrating both the psychiatrically oriented and the AA- and NA-oriented programs. First, psychiatrists must not medicate patients inappropriately. This means that after detoxification, addicts are not to be treated with addictive substances such as barbiturates or benzodiazepines, except in the most extraordinary circumstances. Second, patients with major depressions and other major psychiatric syndromes are to be treated aggressively with nonaddictive psychotropic medications such as tricyclic antidepressants, MAOIs, lithium, or neuroleptics. Usually the benefits of this approach are obvious and will help the patient participate more in AA or other recovery aspects. The biologically and pharmacologically oriented members of the treatment team must soon become aware of the importance of a structured program involving patients and families. Just as the counselor must learn the difference between prescribing diazepam to an alcoholic and prescribing lithium to a manic-depressive addict, so the psychopharmacologist must gain an appreciation of educating a patient about the disease concept of addiction and the need for on-going support systems such as AA and NA. We have found that there is much common ground, particularly with the notion of a disease concept. The disease concept is consistent with notions of biological psychiatry and leads to an emphasis on follow-up treatment. The disease concept also explains the rationale for the professional staff making decisions about treatment that the addict is not suited to make. Certainly the notion that an addict has a biological illness that renders him or her powerless over drug and alcohol use and that requires the addict to "surrender" to a treatment program is acceptable to psychopharmacologists and AA counselors alike.

As mentioned above, the drug-free postdetoxification evaluation period is crucial for assessing treatment needs, including need for psychopharmacology. The need for psychopharmacological treatment of depression is clearer if depressive symptoms persist following detoxification. The lack of a need for psychopharmacological treatment is also more clear if the symptoms are improving spontaneously. In many patients, the model that seems most useful in treatment is simply the two-disease model. That is, a proportion of addicts have major psychiatric disorders just like a proportion of addicts have medical disorders, and they require treatment accordingly. We have found it helpful to suggest that just as in the AA model alcoholism is considered a disease that has a specific treatment, so major depressive illness is a disease in its own right that has its specific treatment. The notion that all depressive symptomatology in an addicted individual is related to the addiction needs to be undercut.

The psychiatrist who is directly involved in treating depression in an addictive population must become familiar with the common manipulations and defenses of the addict, such as denial. The psychiatrist must also become used to being more authoritarian and directive in dealing with the addict and must enlist the patient's family, employer, or others who could influence the patient to stay in treatment. Particularly in the drug addict population, as opposed to the alcoholic, one must be aware of antisocial patterns of behavior.

To monitor the patient's compliance, random supervised blood or urine drug screens are indicated on a regular basis. No psychopharmacologist would want to treat an addict pharmacologically while the addict was self-medicating with street drugs. This not only would color the pharmacological response to prescribed psychotropics and the ability to assess the response, but it might also be medically dangerous because of additive effects. The psychiatrist involved in treating depression in an addict must be aware that, given the relapsing nature of addictions, even if the depression responds to appropriate psychopharmacological treatment there should be no re-laxation in the vigilance over possible relapse into drug and alcohol abuse.

The same basic principles of good psychopharmacological practice that apply to the nonaddicted patient apply to the depressed alcoholic or drug addict. Patients with persistent major depressive illness several weeks after detoxification should be treated pharmacologically with adequate trials of antidepressant medications. Plasma levels of an-tidepressants should be monitored. This is particularly important in addicts and alcoholics because of possible alterations in liver metab-olism of antidepressants as a result of drug effects or possible liver disease. Measuring plasma levels of medications can be especially helpful in monitoring compliance because addicts may be even less compliant than other populations of psychiatric patients. Lithium, MAOI, and the new second-generation antidepressants all could be administered in an addicted population if prescribed appropriately. Possible pressure from an AA or NA group for a recovering alcoholic or addict not to take any prescribed psychotropic medication must also be considered. Patients must be educated very clearly in the two-disease concept and in the need to take psychotropics as well as to participate in appropriate recovery programs.

There may be a small percentage of opioid addicts in whom the best treatment seems to be methadone maintenance (56). We cer-tainly have seen a small fraction of methadone maintenance patients who could not be stabilized with conventional psychiatric treatment, recovery groups, or psychotropic medications after detoxification. Many of these may represent patients with protracted abstinence syndromes. However, the main point is that there is a small per-centage of opioid-addicted patients who may need to return to long-term methadone maintenance as the best symptomatic treatment.

We find the results of integrated, multidisciplinary, tightly struc-tured treatment programs for alcoholics and drug addicts led by psychiatrists encouraging. The outcome data as reported above are encouraging compared to some previous reports in the literature. We feel that psychiatry is on the verge of a new era of recognition of the problems of addiction and sophistication in treating alcoholics and drug addicts. Psychiatry is becoming aware of the need to avoid stereotyping all treatment of these patients and to require indi-vidualization of treatment plans within the context of structured treatment programs emphasizing a lifetime of commitment to re-covery.

A sophisticated integration of psychopharmacological concepts as well as AA concepts will provide a more successful treatment approach to the patient with both addiction and depression or other major psychiatric syndromes. Further understanding of the biological mechanisms of addiction as well as the neurobiological consequences of addiction will also be expected to lead to more successful treatment approaches.

REFERENCES

1. Rounsaville BJ, Weissman MM, Rosenberger PH, et al: Diagnosis and symptoms of depression in opiate addicts: course and relationship to treatment outcome. Arch Gen Psychiatry 39:151–156, 1982

2. Kleber HD, Gold MS: Use of psychotropic drugs in the treatment of methadone maintained narcotic addicts. Ann NY Acad Sci 331:81–98, 1978

3. Dorus W, Senay EC: Depression, demographic dimensions, and drug abuse. Am J Psychiatry 137:699–704, 1980

4. Weissman MM, Pottenger M, Kleber H, et al: Symptom patterns in primary and secondary depression: a comparison of primary depressives with depressed opiate addicts, alcoholics, and schizophrenics. Arch Gen Psychiatry 34:854–862, 1977

5. Rounsaville BJ, Weissman MM, Kleber H, et al: Heterogeneity of psychiatric diagnosis in treated opiate addicts. Arch Gen Psychiatry 39:161–166, 1982

6. Mirin SM, Weiss RD, Sollogub A, et al: Affective illness in substance abusers, in Substance Abuse and Psychopathology. Edited by Mirin SM. Washington, DC, American Psychiatric Press, 1984

7. Dackis CA, Gold MS: Depression in opiate addicts, in Substance Abuse and Psychopathology. Edited by Mirin SM. Washington, DC, American Psychiatric Press, 1984

8. Extein I, Gold MS: Diagnosis and treatment of mood disorders in cocaine abusers. Presented at the annual meeting of National Association of Private Psychiatric Hospitals, Marco Island, Florida, 30 January 1985

9. Cloninger CR, Bohman M, Sigvardsson S: Inheritance of alcohol abuse: cross-fostering analysis of adopted men. Arch Gen Psychiatry, 38:861–868, 1981

10. Khantzian EJ, Khantzian NJ: Cocaine addiction: is there a psychological predisposition? Psychiatric Annals 11:753–759, 1984

11. Robins LN, Helzer JE, Weissman MM: Lifetime prevalence of specific psychiatric disorders in three sites. Arch Gen Psychiatry 41:949–958, 1984

12. American Psychiatric Association: Diagnostic and Statistical Manual of Mental Disorders. 3rd ed. Washington, DC, American Psychiatric Association, 1980

13. Spitzer RL, Endicott J, Robins E: Research Diagnostic Criteria: rationale and reliability. Arch Gen Psychiatry 35:773–782, 1978

14. Dackis CA, Gold MS: Alcoholism, in Advances in Psychopharmacology: Predicting and Improving Treatment Response. Edited by Gold MS, Lydiard RB, Carman JS. Boca Raton, Florida, CRC Press, 1984

15. Alcoholics Anonymous, 3rd ed. New York, Alcoholics Anonymous World Services, 1976

16. Gold MS, Verebey K: The psychopharmacology of cocaine. Psychiatric Annals 14:714–723, 1984

17. Berkow R, Talbolt JH (eds): The Merck Manual of Diagnosis and Therapy. 13th ed. Rahway, New Jersey, Merck & Co, 1977

18. Kleber HD, Riordan CF: The treatment of narcotic withdrawal: a historical review. J Clin Psychiatry 43:30–34, 1982

19. Gold MS, Redmond DE, Kleber HD: Clonidine in opiate withdrawal. Lancet 1:929–930, 1978

20. Mirin SM, Meyer RE, McNamee HB: Psychopathology and mood during heroin use: acute vs. chronic effects. Arch Gen Psychiatry 33:1053–1508, 1976

21. Rounsaville BJ, Kleber HD: Psychiatric disorders and the course of opiate addiction: preliminary findings on predictive significance and diagnostic stability, in Substance Abuse and Psychopathology. Edited by Mirin SM. Washington, DC, American Psychiatric Press, 1984

22. Endicott J, Spitzer RL: A diagnostic interview: the schedule for affective disorders and schizophrenia. Arch Gen Psychiatry 35:837–844, 1978

23. Jaffe JH: Drug addiction and drug abuse, in The Pharmacological Basis of Therapeutics. 6th ed. Edited by Gilman AG, Goodman LS, Gilman A. New York, Macmillan, 1980

24. Ockert DM, Extein I, Gold MS: Variables affecting treatment outcome in middle and upper class opioid and cocaine abusers and addicts. Society for Neuroscience Abstracts 10:1102, 1984

25. Snyder, SH: The opiate receptor and morphine-like peptides in the brain. Am J Psychiatry 135:645–652, 1978

26. Pickar D, Extein I, Gold PW, et al: Endorphins and affective illness, in Endorphins and Opiate Agonists in Psychiatric Research: Clinical Implications. Edited by Shah NS, Donald AS. New York, Plenum Press, 1982

27. Extein I, Pottash ALC, Gold MS, et al: Deficient prolactin response to morphine in depression. Am J Psychiatry 137:845–846, 1980

28. Gold MS, Pottash ALC, Extein I, et al: Anti-endorphin effects of methadone. Lancet 2:972–973, 1980

29. Dackis CA, Gurpegui M, Pottash ALC, et al: Methadone induced hypoadrenalism. Lancet 2:1167, 1982

30. Spensley J: A useful adjunct in the treatment of heroin addicts in a methadone program. Int J Addict 11:191–197, 1976

31. Woody GE, O'Brien CP, Rickels K: Depression and anxiety in heroin addicts: a placebo controlled study of doxepin in combination with methadone. Am J Psychiatry 132:447–450, 1975

32. Kleber HD, Weissman MM, Rounsaville BJ: Imipramine as treatment for depression in addicts. Arch Gen Psychiatry 40:649–653, 1978

33. Woody GE, McLellan AT, Luborsky L, et al: Severity of psychiatric symptoms as a predicator of benefits from psychotherapy: the Veterans Administration–Penn study. Am J Psychiatry 141:1172–1177, 1984

34. Schuckit MA. The clinical implications of primary diagnostic groups among alcoholics. Arch Gen Psychiatry 42:1043–1049, 1985

35. Goodwin DW, Guze SB: Psychiatric Diagnoses. New York, Oxford University Press, 1981

36. Gold MS: 800-COCAINE. New York, Bantam Books, 1984

37. Washton AM, Gold MS: Chronic cocaine abuse: evidence for adverse effects on health and functioning. Psychiatric Annals 14:733–743, 1984

38. VanDyke C, Byck R: Cocaine. Sci Am 246:128–141, 1982

39. Dackis CA, Gold MS: New concepts in cocaine addiction: the dopamine depletion hypothesis. Neurosci Biobehav Rev 9:469–477, 1985

40. Extein I: Brain mechanisms in cocaine dependency, in Cocaine Abuse. Edited by Gold MS, Washton A. New York, Guilford Press (in press)

41. Dackis CA, Estroff TW, Gold MS: Hyperprolactinemia in cocaine abuse. Society for Neuroscience Abstracts 10:1099, 1984

42. Dackis CA, Gold MS: Bromocriptine as treatment of cocaine abuse. Lancet 1:1151–1152, 1985

43. Rosecrans JS: Treatment of cocaine abuse with imipramine, L-tyrosine, and L-tryptophan. Presented at the Seventh World Congress of Psychiatry, Vienna, Austria, July 1983

44. Gawin FH, Kleber HD: Cocaine abuse treatment: open pilot trial with desipramine and lithium carbonate. Arch Gen Psychiatry 41:903–909, 1984

45. Carroll BJ, Feinberg M, Greden JF, et al: A specific laboratory test for the diagnosis of melancholia: standardization, validation and clinical utility. Arch Gen Psychiatry 38:15–22, 1981

46. Smals A, Kloppenberg X: Alcohol-induced pseudo-Cushing's syndrome. Lancet 1:1369, 1977

47. Swartz CM, Dunner FJ: Dexamethasone suppression testing of alcoholics. Arch Gen Psychiatry 39:1309–1312, 1982

48. Dackis CA, Bailey J, Pottash ALC, et al: Specificity of the DST and the TRH test for major depression in alcoholism. Am J Psychiatry 141:680–683, 1984

49. Extein I, Pottash ALC, Gold MS: The thyrotropin-releasing hormone test in the diagnosis of unipolar depression. Psychiatry Res 5:311–316, 1981

50. Loosen PT, Prange AJ: Thyrotropin releasing hormone (TRH): a useful tool for psychoneuroendocrine investigation. Psychoneuroendocrinology 5:63–80, 1980

51. Gold MS, Pottash ALC, Extein I: Hypothyroidism and depression. JAMA 245:1919–1925, 1981

52. Guillemin R, Vargo T, Rossier J, et al: Beta-endorphin and adrenocorticotropin are secreted concomitantly by the pituitary gland. Science 197:1367–1369, 1977

53. Gold PW, Extein I, Pickar D, et al: Suppression of plasma cortisol in depressed patients by acute intravenous methadone infusion. Am J Psychiatry 137:862–863, 1980

54. Martin JB, Reichlan S, Brown EM: Clinical Neuroendocrinology. Philadelphia, FA Davis Co, 1977

55. Dackis CA, Pottash ALC, Gold MS, et al: The dexamethasone suppression test for major depression among opiate addicts. Am J Psychiatry 141:810–811, 1984

56. Dole VP, Nyswander ME, Kreek MJ: Narcotic blockade. Arch Intern Med 118:304–309, 1966

Chapter 7

Medication-Induced and Toxin-Induced Psychiatric Disorders

Todd Wilk Estroff, M.D.
Mark S. Gold, M.D.

Chapter 7

Medication-Induced and Toxin-Induced Psychiatric Disorders

PSYCHIATRIC MISDIAGNOSIS

One of the major advances of psychiatry during the last 10 years has been the growing realization and careful scientific documentation that psychiatric and behavioral symptoms are nonspecific (1–6). As this fact became generally known, ruling out all other possible causes of psychobehavioral symptoms has become a mandatory first step before any definitive psychiatric treatment could begin (1, 3, 4, 6, 7). Whenever this first step in diagnosis is ignored, causative medical illnesses, drug abuse, and medication-induced and toxin-induced psychiatric disorders are often misdiagnosed and mistreated as a primary psychiatric disorder (1–6). Errors of this type can occur among psychiatrists as well as nonpsychiatric physicians for a variety of reasons (6). Unfortunately there are no known pathognomonic signs of medication- and toxin-induced psychiatric disorders based on clinical presentations (Figures 1–9). These disorders must be actively pursued by maintaining a high index of suspicion, carefully reviewing medications, taking a careful environmental toxin history, ordering appropriate laboratory testing, and integrating all of this into a careful diagnostic evaluation of each patient who presents with psychiatric behavioral symptoms. The single fact remains that any symptom can be induced by these disorders and they can easily be misdiagnosed, overlooked, or ignored.

The chances for misdiagnosis are greater today because there has been a massive increase in the development of new drugs in all fields of medicine. Most of these drugs were developed within the last 50 years, but the greatest percentage were introduced within the last 30 years. These new drugs have contributed to the reporting of psychiatric side effects (8, 9). In addition, greater physician awareness of these possible reactions has played a part in a general increase in the documentation of drug-induced psychiatric side effects.

Poorly Studied Field

This area of overlap psychiatry and medicine is so complicated that exact or even approximate values for the incidence and prevalence of medication- and toxin-induced psychiatric complications are not precisely known. Only rough outdated estimates exist. This chapter is intended to review as completely as possible the psychiatric complications and side effects of medications and toxins as well as provide some general guidelines to the evaluation and treatment of these disorders.

Much of the evidence cited in this chapter is based on single case reports, which may not be totally accurate. Several problems occur when case reports are relied on too heavily. Many of the reports originate from nonpsychiatrists who have little or no training in the accurate performance and documentation of a mental status examination. A patient demonstrating behavioral symptoms such as extreme panic, agitation, hallucinations, or catatonia is often labeled as being "psychotic" or "schizophrenic" when this clearly is not the case. Frequently there is enough case material in the case report to document an acute delirious or toxic state that has been misdiagnosed.

Even when reports are made by psychiatrists, many diagnoses made prior to 1980 are not based on the clearly defined and systemized criteria found in the Research Diagnostic Criteria (RDC) (9a) or the *Diagnostic and Statistical Manual of Mental Disorders*, Third Edition (DSM-III) (7) and are therefore less reliable.

Additional problems occur when psychiatric reactions are reported after a single dose of medication has been given. However, single-dose trials must remain suspect because they do not take other intercurrent variables into account. Causality is inferred by the clearing of symptoms. While this can be highly suggestive, the patient is never rechallenged with the offending agent, using either the A, B, AB, or ABA designs so critical to careful scientific inquiry.

One other method that can help document causality is by demonstrating simultaneous toxic blood levels and the presence of psychiatric symptoms that resolve as soon as they drop to the therapeutic levels.

Typical autopsy or pathological brain morphologic changes such as those seen in the basal ganglia manganese poisoning or diffuse hypoxic damage can be helpful in proving a causal relationship.

Few Epidemiologic Studies

The area of medication and psychobehavioral side effects has been largely ignored in epidemiologic studies, although a few exist. The Boston Collaborative Drug-Related Program (10) has documented

2.7 percent psychiatric and behavioral reaction in 9,000 patients. Other studies have looked at large numbers of patients taking antiparkinsonian agents (11) and antihypertensive agents for psychiatric side effects (12, 13) and are discussed in more detail later in this chapter. Whenever information about percentages of side effects is known, it is documented within the text in parentheses.

Other problems can arise in these epidemiologic studies if there is no comparison between the observed rates and the natural incidence and prevalence of these disorders in the normal population. Likewise it is important to choose appropriate control groups (14).

Types of Reactions

In addition, it is important to define as precisely as possible the type of reaction that has occurred. If the psychiatric symptoms are caused totally by the offending agent and they disappear as it is eliminated from the patient's body, the relationship would be termed a causal one (4, 6). LSD hallucinosis is a good example of this situation. On the other hand, if the agent interacts with a latent psychiatric predisposition and psychiatric symptoms persist, it is termed an exacerbating reaction (4, 6). Reserpine-induced depression in an individual who has already had a major depression is a good example.

Other reactions can be classified as immediate, as in an idiosyncratic reaction or an overdose, or they may be delayed as the result of the build up of multiple doses over a long period of time. If given in high enough doses, some medications will produce symptoms even in normal individuals (15–17). Synergistic reactions can occur only when two agents are used in combination but would not occur with either agent alone (14). Lastly, there is also a class of psychiatric symptoms that occur only during withdrawal in a dependent individual (8, 18–22). These symptoms will often remit on administration of the tolerated agent as occurs during alcohol, diazepam (Valium), barbiturate, or other seductive hypnotic withdrawal.

Individuals at Risk

The individuals most at risk for the development of psychiatric symptoms side effects (sometimes labeled idiosyncratic) are those who already have some impairment of cognitive processes, such as the elderly or the mentally retarded. Medically ill individuals are also more prone to develop psychiatric side effects. They can have compromised functioning of a critical organ system that is responsible for normal drug metabolism. For example, when kidney or liver failure occur, drug or toxins levels may rise, causing toxic blood levels that can result in increased psychiatric mobidity (14). Individuals under medical supervision also tend to be on multiple medications contributing to the risk of synergistic reaction. Of course, individuals with brain tumors, epilepsy, trauma, anoxic central nervous system (CNS) damage, or previous major psychiatric illnesses are at higher risk.

Any individual who is suspected of having any of these preexisting risk factors must be carefully evaluated. All medication should be stopped if possible. If it is not possible, an effective medication with fewer psychiatric side effects should be substituted during evaluation (4, 6).

PRESCRIBED MEDICATIONS

Psychiatric Medications (Figure 1)

Tricyclic Antidepressants. Antidepressants can cause immediate toxic effects or interact with an individual patient's underlying psychopathology. Immediate toxic effects include visual hallucinations, urinary retention, increased temperature, tachycardia, mydriasis, dry mouth, dry or flushed skin color, paralytic ileus, convulsions, coma, and delirium (5). Many of these signs and symptoms are caused by the tricyclic's anticholinergic properties, making it difficult to distinguish from atropine, antihistamines, belladonna alkaloids, antipsychotics, certain plants, benztropine, and trihexphenidyl overdoses. Quantitative blood testing can help diagnose a suspected overdose, either intentional or accidental. Tricyclic delirium may be reversed by i.v. physostigmine (23), but it is not a general antidote. Patients with a bipolar vulnerability who present as a major depression can be switched into mania or have a psychotic episode when they are treated with tricyclics (5). Antidepressants can cause a schizophrenic patient to become more psychotic (24).

Similar psychotic reactions have been reported for tetracyclics monoamine oxidase inhibitors, and other antidepressants (25). With-

Medication	Psychosis	Mania	Depression	Organic	Hallucinations	Others
Antidepressants Tricyclic	XX	XX		XX	Visual	
Antidepressants MAOI	XX	XX				Anxiety, nervousness, agitation, insomnia
Antipsychotics	XX		XX	XX		Oversedation, total mute, malignant syndrome
Lithium			XX	XX		
Sed / Hypnotics Benzodiazepines	XX		XX			Oversedation, disinhibition
Disulfiram	XX	XX	XX	XX		Anxiety

Figure 1. Psychiatric Medications

drawal symptoms similar to those of influenza with insomnia, nausea, and vomiting occur in adults on 150 + mg of tricyclics per day. This occurs much more frequently in children (5, 26).

Monoamine Oxidase Inhibitor Antidepressants. Monoamine oxidase inhibitors can induce behavioral side effects similar to other antidepressants but are more likely to induce manic symptoms because they are structurally related to epinephrine and amphetamine. Anxiety, nervousness, agitation, insomnia, and euphoria can progress into symptoms indistinguishable from DSM-III mania or schizophrenia (26). Overdoses, toxic interactions, idiosyncratic interactions, and tyramine crisis are also described (5, 27).

Antipsychotics. Antipsychotics including phenothiazines, butyrophenones, thioxanthenes, molindone, and loxapine can produce psychiatric side effects ranging from oversedation to total mutism (28) as well as severe catatonia (29, 30). Parkinsonism and covert and withdrawal emergent dyskinesias, especially in children, are reported in addition to tardive dyskinesia (31). Akathisia and akinesia can often be misdiagnosed as anxiety and depression (5, 32). Neuroleptic malignant syndrome is a rare, severe toxic syndrome that produces fever, muscular rigidity, akinesia, severe delirium, and elevated creatine phosphokinase levels (5, 33, 34). This condition resembles malignant hyperthermia.

The combination of antipsychotics with other drugs possessing anticholinergic properties can be synergistic, causing an anticholinergic delerium that may be misinterpreted as a worsening of the psychosis (35).

Nausea, vomiting, diarrhea, perspiration, restlessness, insomnia, shivering, headaches, increased appetite, and giddiness (31) can occur when these medications are discontinued and as part of a neuroleptic withdrawal syndrome.

Lithium Carbonate. Toxic lithium levels can cause decreased concentration, increased depression, and a toxic delirium, especially if they are not monitored carefully. It is fortunately an uncommon phenomenon (36–38). Suicide attempts have resulted in permanent neurotoxic damage caused by elevated serum lithium levels (39, 40).

Benzodiazepines and Other Sedative-Hypnotics. Benzodiazepines and other sedative-hypnotics can produce oversedation and disinhibition while the drug is taken. Rare reports of severe depression with suicidal ideation, as well as depersonalization and frank psychosis, have been noted (35). The elderly are most vulnerable to this kind of delirium. Psychiatric misdiagnoses occur, most commonly when psychiatric symptoms occur and are not recognized during withdrawal in dependent individuals (8, 18–22).

Disulfiram (Antabuse).   Disulfiram is often used in the treatment of alcoholism. It causes the severe reactions of nausea and vomiting when abstinence is broken and alcohol (ethanol) is ingested. Psychiatric symptoms include anxiety and severe depression. The disulfiram psychoses are indistinguishable from DSM-III bipolar mania and schizophrenia (9, 41–44). Delirium can develop with or without associated psychiatric symptoms. Disulfiram and its major metabolites inhibit both dopamine beta hydroxylase and porphyrin metabolism, which could account for the etiology of the psychiatric effects. Treatment consists of withdrawal of the disulfiram and use of minor tranquilizers. Antipsychotic medications worsen the symptoms and are therefore contraindicated (9, 43, 44).

Antihypertensive Medication (Figure 2)

Reserpine.   Reserpine has long been noted to induce depression. Other antihypertensives can precipitate depression, but less frequently than reserpine. Patients who have a prior history of depression and who have been treated with more than 0.5 mg/day for at least 2 to 8 months are the most vulnerable to reserpine-induced depression (12, 45–49). Reserpine can also produce acute confusional states with psychotic features (49) as well as serve as an antipsychotic in refractory psychoses.

Alpha-Methyl Dopa.   Alpha-methyl dopa acts as a false neurotransmitter peripherally and has a prominent CNS action. When data from 2,320 patients from 65 studies were compiled, psychiatric side effects included sleep disorders (0.8 percent), dreams and nightmares (1.9 percent), and depression (3.6 percent) (13). Rare organic toxic states with paranoia or psychosis have been reported (13, 50). More depression was reported in past years when higher dosages of alpha-methyl dopa were used.

Medication	Psychosis	Mania	Depression	Organic	Hallucinations	Others
Reserpine	XX		XX	XX		
α-Methyl Dopa	XX		XX	XX		Nightmares, disordered sleep
Clonidine	XX	XX	XX			Sedation, fatigue, anxiety
Propranolol			XX		Hypnagogic Hypnopompic	Nightmares, fatigue
Guanethidine						
Debrisoquine						
Bethanidine						
Hydralazine						
Minoridyl						
Diuretics						

Figure 2.   Antihypertensive Medications

Clonidine. Clonidine is a centrally acting α_2 agonist. Review of 791 patients treated for hypertension with clonidine revealed frequent sedation and fatigue (47.6 percent), some sleep disturbance (4.7 percent), and little depression (1.5 percent). There are rare reports of nervousness, irritability, paranoia, and hypomania (13). The first signs of clonidine abuse or overdose can be psychomotoric retardation, decreased temperature, bradycardia, miosis, paralytic ileus, and coma.

Propranolol (Inderal). Propranolol is a beta-blocking agent with both central and peripheral actions. It is used for a wide variety of disorders in addition to control of hypertension. In 4,708 cases, it was reported to cause drowsiness and fatigue (3.1 percent), sleep disorders (0.4 percent), increased dreams and nightmares (1 percent), predominantly hypnagogic and hypnopompic hallucinations (0.5 percent), and depression (0.7 percent) (13).

Other Antihypertensive Agents. Guanethidine, debrisoquine, bethanidine, hydralazine, minoridyl, and all diuretics have yet to show any convincing evidence that they produce any major psychiatric side effects (13).

Cardiovascular Medications (Figure 3)

Antiarrhythmic Drugs. Lidocaine (51) and procainamide (52) have been reported to cause psychosis, especially in the intensive care unit setting. McCrum and Guidry (52) report a case in which procainamide repeatedly induced a manic or schizoaffective episode in a 45-year-old man previously diagnosed and treated as having a bipolar disorder.

Disopyramide causes an acute transient toxic psychosis with delusions of persecution and auditory and visual hallucinations (53–55). These symptoms may be due to its anticholinergic properties.

Digitalis. Duroziez first described "delire digitalique" in 1874 (56). Since then mental symptoms have often been noted as the first and only sign of digitalis intoxication. The causal link was proven when it was demonstrated that psychiatric symptoms corresponded to toxic levels. These symptoms can also occur in association with the other

Medication	Psychosis	Mania	Depression	Organic	Hallucinations	Others
Lidocaine	XX					
Procainamide	XX	XX				
Disopyramide	XX				Auditory and Visual	
Digitalis	XX			XX	Auditory and Visual	Mutism, labile mood swings

Figure 3. Cardiovascular Medications

well-documented toxic symptoms of digitalis toxicity such as arrhythmia, nausea, vomiting, and yellow-tinted vision.

Death can result if digitalis toxicity is misdiagnosed and mistreated psychiatrically as a "coronary care unit psychosis" (57). The psychiatric symptoms can include visual or auditory hallucinations (58–60), paranoid ideation (58–61), thought disorder, mutism, and labile mood swings (61). This can occur in clear consciousness, but frequently there is some degree of disorientation or agitation. All of these mental symptoms clear when the serum levels fall from the toxic range into the therapeutic range.

Neurological Disorder Medications (Figure 4)

Anticonvulsant Medications. Epileptic patients have a higher incidence of associated psychiatric disturbance even without medication and psychiatric symptoms can increase with the addition of even one medication. Many patients are often on two or more anticonvulsants at a time and are thus at higher risk for synergistic side effects. Confusional states, including sedation, mood changes, fluctuating energy levels (62–64), excitement, irritability, tearfulness, aggression, and hyperactivity, can occur among patients taking anticonvulsant medications. Psychotic features can include somatic and paranoid delusions and auditory, visual, and tactile hallucinations that are indistinguishable from schizophrenia or mania. Anticonvulsants can also cause acute delirium.

Phenytoin (Dilantin, Diphenylhydantoin). Phenytoin has been called the "digitalis of neurology" because of its widespread use for seizure control. It can also be used for ventricular arrhythmias. Acute delir-

Medication	Psychosis	Mania	Depression	Organic	Hallucinations	Others
Phenytoin	XX			XX	Visual and Tactile	Somatic delusions
Barbiturates			XX	XX		Tearful, hyperactive, aggression in children
Primidone	XX	XX		XX		Mood swings, paranoia, personality changes
Ethosuximide	XX	XX	XX		XX	Anxiety, aggression, night terrors, lethargy
Carbamazepine	XX					Anxiety, restlessness, drowsiness
Baclofen	XX	XX	XX		Auditory and Visual	
L-dopa	XX	XX	XX	XX	Auditory and Visual	Vivid dreams, illusions
Bromocriptine	XX	XX		XX	Auditory, Visual, and Olfactory	Vivid dreams
Anticholinergics	XX			XX		

Figure 4. Neurological Medications

ium with hallucinations, encephalopathy, tactile and visual hallucinations (63, 65), somatic delusions, and schizophrenic-like psychoses
(62, 63) can occur. Acute overdose may produce nystagmus, vertigo,
increased tendon reflexes, muscular rigidity, slurred speech, drowsiness, confusion, psychomotoric activation, and hallucinations. All
signs and symptoms are directly related to blood level (e.g., nystagmus, 20 μg/ml; ataxia, 30 μg/ml; drowsiness, 40 μg/ml).

Barbiturates. Barbiturates can cause different psychiatric side effects in adults and children. Confusional states, drowsiness, sedation,
and depression occur in adults, whereas excitement, irritability, tearfulness, aggression, and a hyperkinetic syndrome occur most commonly in children (62, 63). Misdiagnosis of barbiturate tolerance
and withdrawal states is common. This is especially unfortunate because the psychiatric side effects of barbiturates and most other sedative-hypnotics occur during withdrawal in addicted individuals.

Primidone. Primidone is not a barbiturate but has a similar structure and is metabolized into phenobarbital. It is therefore not surprising to find a spectrum of side effects similar to those of barbiturates, including excess sedation, confusional states, major mood
swings, paranoid and confusional psychosis (62, 63), and personality
changes (66).

Ethosuximide. Ethosuximide is used primarily in the treatment of
petit mal epilepsy and is thus more commonly used in children and
young adults. Anxiety, depression, delusions, hallucinations, psychosis (67, 68), lethargy, and euphoria (63) as well as night terrors,
aggression, and paranoia are included in the wide continuum of
psychiatric symptoms seen in this population (62).

Carbamazepine (Tegretol). Carbamazepine's psychiatric manifestations are seldom noted but can include drowsiness, anxiety, restlessness, and rare reports of worsening an active psychosis (62, 63,
69).

Most of the side effects of phenytoin, barbiturates, primidone,
ethosuximide, and carbamazepine are associated with elevated blood
levels and clear in a short period of days to a week when the offending
agent is stopped and blood level closely monitored. Idiosyncratic
reactions at therapeutic levels are known to occur.

Baclofen (Lioresal). Baclofen is a muscle relaxant that is structurally
similar to γ-aminobutyric acid (GABA) and presumably acts by inhibiting GABA-mediated spinal reflexes. Jones and Lance (70) reported prominent psychiatric side effects in 113 patients treated with
baclofen. Symptoms included hallucinations, illusions, paranoia, euphoria, aphrodisiac affects, depression, anxiety, and a suicide attempt.
The side effects usually subsided within 24 hours. Paranoid ideation,

agitation, hallucinations, and urinary retention have been reported by Skausig and Korsgaard (71). They also reported that baclofen induced the depressed phase of a bipolar illness in another patient. Paranoid ideation, auditory and visual hallucinations, and DSM-III mania have been reported when baclofen was stopped; these were cleared when medication was restarted (72, 73).

L-Dopa. In a review (11) of 908 parkinsonian patients in 20 separate studies, L-dopa caused a 20 percent rate of psychiatric symptoms. The symptoms included confusion or delirium (4.4 percent); depression (4.2 percent); agitation or activation (3.6 percent); psychosis, delusions, or paranoia (3.6 percent); hypomania (1.5 percent); hypersexuality (0.9 percent); and other symptoms (1.5 percent). Similar results were reported in 126 patients treated for more than 1 year (74). Patients with previous psychiatric symptoms as well as dementia and postencephalitic parkinsonism were at much higher risk to develop these symptoms. Moskovitz et al. (75) actively excluded the three "at risk" subpopulations of parkinsonian patients and still found very high rates of psychiatric symptoms in a sample of 88 patients treated with L-dopa. The symptoms included vivid dreams (30.7 percent), hallucinations (mostly visual) (29.5 percent), illusions (5.7 percent), and psychosis (12.5 percent). Interestingly, 9.1 percent of these patients exhibited no confusion whereas 3.4 percent demonstrated some organicity.

Bromocriptine. Bromocriptine has recently been introduced into clinical medicine for the treatment of parkinsonism because of its ability to stimulate dopamine production in the brain. It is an amide of lysergic acid but it is not pharmacologically a hallucinogen like LSD (a diethylamide of lysergic acid), except possibly in very high doses (76, 77). Calne et al. (78) reported psychiatric disturbance severe enough to force discontinuation of bromocriptine in 8 (8.7 percent) of 92 patients treated with high doses for 6 months or longer. The structural relationship to LSD may account for the auditory, visual, and olfactory hallucinations that were noted as well as confusion, vivid dreams, and paranoid delusions. It has also been reported to cause mania (79). The psychiatric symptoms, when they occur, are more prolonged than with L-dopa (78, 79).

Anticholinergic Agents. Anticholinergic antiparkinsonian agents such as benztropine (Cogentin), trihexphenidyl (Artane), and procyclidine (Kemadrin) are used in the treatment of naturally occurring and medication-induced Parkinson's disease. They can cause a classic atropine, anticholinergic psychosis. A toxic psychosis occurs and is capable of mimicking any psychiatric syndrome. In most cases it is actually an acute delirium that is limited to the time course of the drug's action and clears rapidly. Psychosis can be produced in any individual if a large enough dose is given. This dose is reported to be 10 mg of atropine or its equivalent in adults (80). There are no reports of prolonged psychosis after the acute effects wear off. The psychosis is also rapidly reversible when physostigmine is given i.v. Other cholinesterase inhibitors do *not* reverse the CNS toxicity of atropinic anticholinergic compounds because they are not tertiary amines like physostigmine and therefore do not cross the blood-brain barrier.

Unusual sources of anticholinergic poisoning include eating the flowers of *Datura stromonium* (e.g., Jimson weed, angels trumpet, devils trumpet) for psychedelic effects (81), atropinic eye drops, pre-op medication with atropine and scopolamine, or intentional poisoning in which ophthalmologic eye drops are instilled into an unsuspecting victim's drink in a bar as a cruel joke or to facilitate robbery by disorienting the victim (82).

Gastrointestinal Medications (Figure 5)

Cimetidine. Cimetidine is an histamine H_2 receptor blocker used in the treatment of gastric hypersecretion disorders including duodenal ulcers. It can cause mild symptoms of acute mental confusion (113–117) as well as a more severe syndrome consisting of confusion, agitation, and auditory and visual hallucinations, which clears 1 to 2 days after the cimetidine is stopped (118–121). Bizarre speech, fluctuating levels of consciousness (120), and extreme paranoia can also appear in certain individuals (119). Agarwal (116) reported a

Medication	Psychosis	Mania	Depression	Organic	Hallucinations	Others
GASTROINTESTINAL MEDICATIONS						
Cimetidine	XX		XX	XX	Auditory and Visual	
OVER-THE-COUNTER MEDICATIONS						
Phenyl-propanolamine	XX		XX			
Ephedrine	XX		XX			
Pseudephedrine	XX		XX			
Aminophylline	XX		XX			
NONSTEROIDAL ANTIINFLAMMATORY MEDICATIONS						
Indomethacin	XX		XX		XX	Anxiety, agitation, hostile, depersonalization
Sulindac	XX		XX			Angry, combative, homicidal, obsessive talking

Figure 5. Gastrointestinal, Over-the-Counter, and Nonsteroidal Anti-inflammatory Medications

case in which visual hallucinations alone occurred, followed by amnesia. Jefferson (122) documented a case of depression with clear consciousness caused by cimetidine therapy. These mental changes are more prone to occur in the elderly, the seriously ill, and especially among alcoholics with liver damage (118, 121).

Over-the-Counter Medications (Figure 5)

Stimulant over-the-counter medications containing phenylpropanolamine, ephedrine, pseudoephedrine, and aminophylline have been noted to induce psychosis and depression in a small segment of the population.

Nonsteroidal Antiinflammatory Medications (Figure 5)

Indomethacin (Indocin) and sulindac (clinoril) are structurally similar nonsteroidal antiinflammatory agents. Both have been reported to cause psychiatric symptoms after only one dose. Indomethacin has been reported to produce anxiety, agitation, hostility, paranoia, depersonalization, depression, hallucinations, and psychosis (83–87).

Sulindac, in as little as one 50-mg dose, was suspected as causing bizarre behavior, obsessive talking, delusions, paranoia, and combative behavior (88). Thornton (89) reported irritability, depression, paranoia, angry outbursts, and homicidal threats within 48 hours of starting sulindac. All symptoms resolved promptly on discontinuation of the sulindac or indomethacin.

Anticancer Medications (Figure 6)

Corticosteroids. Corticosteroids, especially prednisone, are frequently used in the treatment of various forms of cancer. They are well known to produce the psychiatric disorders indistinguishable from any RDC disorder from depression to mania and including schizophreniform psychoses (6).

Medication	Psychosis	Mania	Depression	Organic	Hallucinations	Others
Steroids	XX	XX	XX			
Decarbazine		XX	XX			
Hexamethylamine		XX	XX	XX		
Methotrexate				XX		
5 - FU				XX		Labile mood
Vincristine		XX	XX	XX		
Vinblastine		XX				Anxiety
Mithramycin						Agitation, anxiety, irritable
Asparaginase		XX	XX			Personality changes
Procarbazine		XX				Drowsiness

Figure 6. Anticancer Medications

Alkylating Agents (Decarbazine and Hexamethylamine). Decarbazine and hexamethylamine are alkylating agents, both of which are reported to produce psychiatric side effects. Confusion and depression were reported in 5 percent of patients treated with decarbazine (90). Confusion, depression, hallucinations, and suicide attempts were reported in 20 percent of patients treated with hexamethylamine (90, 91).

Methotrexate. A multifocal leukoencephalopathy accompanied by confusion, tremor, ataxia, irritability, and somnolence can occur in methotrexate-treated patients. There are electroencephalogram (EEG) abnormalities associated with affected areas of the temporal and parietal lobes. Folic acid treatment can help stabilize and sometimes help reverse the leukoencephalopathy (92).

5-Fluorouracil (5-FU). 5-Fluorouracil (5-FU) treatment can cause decreased concentration, mood lability, and a parkinsonism syndrome when given in i.v. doses of 5 mg/kg. Symptoms usually reverse several weeks after the last dose (90).

Vinca Alkaloids (Vincristine and Vinblastine). Vincristine given in doses 75 μg/kg and higher is well known to be a neurotoxin (90). Late occurring irritability, depression, and hallucinations are reported as well as seizures and coma. Vinblastine produces anxiety and depression in 80 percent of patients within 2 to 3 days after treatment.

Mithramycin. Increasing agitation, anxiety, and irritability have developed during treatment with mithramycin.

L-Asparaginase. All patients treated with L-asparaginase showed EEG changes at the same time they developed confusion, delirium, stupor, personality changes, and severe depression (93–95). No manic or schizophreniform episodes have been reported (90).

Other Anticancer Agents. Procarbazine, another monoamine oxidase inhibitor, is reported as causing manic episodes (96) as well as drowsiness to stupor along with slowing of the EEG. Mitotane has been reported to cause confusional states.

Anesthetic Medications (Figure 7)

Immediate Reactions to Preanesthetics. Certain preanesthetics have been found to cause mild to severe psychiatric and behavioral symptoms immediately after administration and before general anesthetics are given. Nalorphine caused feelings of suffocation, panic, fear of impending death, delusions, and auditory and visual hallucinations. Levorphan produced "queer behavior" and fear; pentazocine can induce overactive, rambling, or "crazy" thoughts and fear of dying (97). Preanesthetics have also been associated with postanesthetic excitement, especially when atropine or scopolamine are used as

preanesthetics. When they were used in combination with a barbiturate, psychiatric symptoms were even more frequent (98).
General Anesthetic Agents. The greatest amounts of postanesthetic excitement occurs when cyclopropane and ether are used for general anesthesia (98). Halothane and isoflurane anesthesia can produce psychiatric symptoms, which peak 2 days after general anesthesia and resolves by the 30th day. Fatigue, depression, confusion, anger, tension, and corresponding decreases in friendliness and vigor (99) have all been noted.

Antibiotic Medications (Figure 8)

Antituberculosis Agents. Iproniazid is a monoamine oxidase inhibitor used to treat tuberculosis. It was clear from its first clinical use that this medication could elevate patients' moods (100). The changes noted ranged from mild increases in mood, through mania, to psychosis with either paranoid hallucinations or organic brain syndromes.

Isoniazid is not a monoamine oxidase inhibitor but is similar to both iproniazid and niacin in chemical structure. It has caused delirium (9) and toxic psychoses. Irritability, paranoid ideation, thought disorder, and auditory and visual hallucinations with either a clear or clouded consciousness, have also been observed (9, 101–104). There is some evidence that cute pellagra (niacin deficiency) was precipitated by isoniazid therapy. This resulted in a catatonic, depressed state with a gross thought disorder and refusal to eat, which responded to therapy with nicotinic acid (105). Although there are several reports (9, 102–104) of prolonged or residual symptoms, most cases of isoniazid-induced psychiatric symptoms clear rapidly when the isoniazid is stopped.
Cycloserine. Cycloserine is usually used in combination with other drugs to treat tuberculosis. When it has been used as the sole medication, nervousness, irritability, anxiety, confusion, paranoid delu-

Medication	Psychosis	Mania	Depression	Organic	Hallucinations	Others
Nalorphine	XX				Auditory and Visual	Panic, suffocation, fear of impending death
Levorphan						Fear, "queer behavior"
Atropine						Postanesthetic excitement
Scopolamine						Postanesthetic excitement
Cyclopropane						Postanesthetic excitement
Halothane			XX	XX		Anger, tension, fatigue
Isoflurane			XX	XX		Anger, tension, fatigue
Pentazocine						Overactive, rambling crazy thoughts, fear of dying

Figure 7. Anesthetic Medications

sions, and hallucinations with or without delirium developed. These symptoms become increasingly severe as serum levels rise. Other cycloserine-induced syndromes have included depression, mania, schizophrenic reactions, and toxic psychoses (9, 104, 106).

Procaine Penicillin G. Intramuscular procaine penicillin G can cause brief but such severe psychiatric symptoms that the patient appears psychotic. Disorientation, extreme agitation, and ideas of impending doom can occur along with hallucinations and gross thought disorder. Some patients appear to be manic. Grand mal seizures also have been reported (107–109). This reaction does not occur with any other forms of penicillin and it is not an allergic phenomenon. The procaine is probably the causative agent because toxic levels have been documented at the same time as the psychiatric symptoms. Within 10 to 30 minutes the serum procaine level falls to nontoxic levels and there is a rapid resolution of all psychiatric symptoms (109).

Amphotericin B. Amphotericin B administered intrathecally to a patient with coccidioidal meningitis caused an acute toxic delirium with corresponding EEG changes, which resolved when the dosage was reduced (110).

Chloroquine and Quinacrine. Chloroquine is an antimalarial and antiamebic agent. It is also used for a variety of dermatological problems. Quinacrine is a related compound used for the treatment of *Giardia* and tapeworm infestations. Both are known to produce a rapidly reversible psychosis consisting of hallucinations and manic and delusional features (111, 112).

Heavy Metals and Toxins (Figure 9)

Many aspects of poisoning with heavy metals are well known and are the subject of readily available, excellent, comprehensive discussions. Psychiatric complications of heavy metals deserves special emphasis because even when the existence of toxicity is appreciated,

Medication	Psychosis	Mania	Depression	Organic	Hallucinations	Others
Iproniazid	XX	XX		XX	XX	
Isoniazid	XX		XX	XX	Auditory and Visual	Catatonia
Cycloserine	XX	XX	XX	XX	XX	Nervousness, irritability, anxiety
Procaine Penicillin G	XX	XX		XX	XX	Extreme agitation, fear of impending death
Amphotericin B				XX		
Chloroquine	XX	XX			XX	
Quinacrine	XX	XX			XX	

Figure 8. Antibiotic Medications

information is often insufficient as to how those materials affect the brain functioning and psychiatric status.

Many heavy metals are so essential to health that deficiency diseases can result if there is not enough of the metal present in an individual body. Heavy metals have a high specific gravity of 5.0 or more. Metals are not degradable and can combine with other molecules in forming toxic organo metals. They include iron, copper, zinc, manganese, chromium, nickel, magnesium, molybdenum, cobalt, strontium, vanadium, and selenium. Among the heavy metals considered highly toxic to humans are lead, antimony, beryllium, cadmium, and mercury. Aluminum has, in the past, been though inert and nontoxic but it is now documented as the toxic agent in dialysis dementia.

Lead. Although lead poisoning has been well known for more than 2,000 years, much debate about lead poisoning has centered on how to measure it. There are currently four different ways to measure: in blood, bone (teeth), urine, and hair specimens. In the past, blood levels above 60 μg/dl in adults were universally acknowledged to be toxic (38, 123), but these levels were recently lowered to 40 μg/dl (124, 125).

Because the brain is the least forgiving organ, the lower limit of lead toxicity is constantly being lowered as more and more subtle

Substance	Psychosis	Mania	Depression	Organic	Hallucinations	Others
Lead			XX	XX		Lower IQ and hyperactivity in children
Mercury	XX		XX	XX		Extreme anxiety, strange form of Xenophobia
Arsenic	XX	XX	XX	XX	Visual	
Manganese	XX	XX	XX			Destruction of nigro striatum
Bismuth	XX		XX	XX	Visual	Anxiety
Thallium	XX		XX	XX		
Aluminum			XX	XX	XX	
Tin (Organo)			XX			Unprovoked rage attacks
Magnesium	XX		XX	XX		
Copper	XX	XX	XX	XX	XX	
Vanadium	??		XX			
Cadmium						Associated with learning disabilities in children
Bromine	XX	XX	XX	XX	Auditory and Visual	
Anticholinergics	XX		XX	XX		Prominent anxiety
Carbon Monoxide	XX		XX	XX		Catatonia, borderline personality, panic attack
Carbon Dioxide						Precipitate panic attack
Volatile Hydrocarbons		XX	XX	XX	Auditory and Visual	Conduct disorder, panic anxiety, personality change

Figure 9. Heavy Metals and Toxins

CNS and psychiatric symptoms are monitored and clearly defined as earlier stages of lead toxicity, which occur before frank encephalopathy and seizures develop or other organ systems are affected. This readjustment of normal ranges occurred when cognitive, mood, behavioral, and psychiatric symptoms were defined as toxic symptoms.

Even this lowering of "normal values" may not be enough because, when IQs's are measured in children, lead levels above 13 μg/dl are associated with impaired performance. Obviously much more research in this area is needed to establish safe normal values (126).

Many authors object to the use of blood levels of lead because they claim it reflects only recent exposure and does not accurately portray total body lead burden. However, blood lead levels have been shown to be stable over a period of 3 to 6 months (127). Total body lead level can also be estimated by analyzing bone lead levels. This can be easily estimated in children when their deciduous teeth (bone) are shed to make room for adult teeth.

Urinary lead levels are also reported to reflect the total body lead burden. Lead levels between 0.15 and 0.20 mg/L are reported toxic in adults in the urine (3) of untreated individuals. After administration of 250 mg of penicillamine (128, 129), greater than 0.08 mg/L of lead is considered toxic, while after im administration of 1 g of EDTA (124), 1000 μg/24 or more is reported as an abnormal level.

Hair lead levels can also be measured. Pubic hair is preferred since it is most protected from external lead contamination.

Lead poisoning is especially prone to having associated psychiatric symptoms because the biochemical malfunction it causes is similar in many respects to porphyria (123). In children evidence is mounting that increased lead levels, no matter what the source, or how it is measured, is associated with the symptoms of hyperactivity (128–130) and lower intellectual functioning (126, 131).

In adults Baker et al. (125) have demonstrated that as brief an exposure to sources of lead as 3 months can cause tension, fatigue, confusion, anger, and depression in a dose-related fashion between 40 and 60 μg/dl of serum. These progressive changes are reversible when exposure is discontinued. Of all patients with documented lead poisoning, 13 percent had an initial complaint of depression (124). When a psychiatric examination was performed, 22.6 percent were found to be depressed with vegetative signs.

Mercury. Exposure to mercury can occur in three different forms. The kind of exposure has major implications as to how rapidly psychiatric symptoms develop because elemental mercury ingestion results in brain concentrations 10 times greater than occurs after exposure to inorganic or organic mercury molecules (3).

Mercury-related psychiatric symptoms have been known for centuries, especially among felt makers in the fur-cutting trade (132) who had heavy mercury vapor exposure. This is possibly the source of the expression "mad as a hatter."

The psychiatric symptoms of mercury poisoning include mood changes, severe irritability (44.2 percent), anxiety, psychomotor retardation, prominent depression (74.4 percent), and a unique form of xenophobia in which patients avoid contact with strangers. They are also so self-conscious that they are unable to function under any form of direct supervision (133). The poisoning is related to the blood level, will progress, and will result in a permanent dementia if the source of the insult is not identified and eliminated.

Arsenic. Arsenic may be absorbed systematically from antiamoebic antibiotics, insect and rat poisons, and homemade alcoholic beverages. It can be ingested accidentally in children or deliberately as part of a suicide or homicide attempt.

Acute massive ingestions can result in death within a few hours (3, 134), but commonly symptoms start with a feeling of burning in the throat, difficulty swallowing, nausea, vomiting, severe abdominal pain, and rice water diarrhea. Mania, delirium, and coma can accompany cyanosis and a garlic smell.

Arsenic poisoning most often causes a peripheral neuropathy but the CNS is selectively affected in as many as 10 percent of cases (135, 136). Other symptoms can include seizures, heart failure, edema, anorexia, weight loss, anergia, and myelopathy and they can progress to toxic delirium characterized by confusion, disorientation, crying, agitation, depression, emotional lability, paranoid and delusional ideation, and visual hallucinations. All of these can be confused with a Korsakoff's psychosis (135–138).

Finding hair loss, skin thickening, increased pigmentation, and a tranverse white line across the nails can help make a diagnosis, but it must be confirmed by measuring blood and urine levels for arsenic.

Manganese. Various terms have been applied to the psychiatric symptoms that develop in persons exposed to manganese. It has been variously called manganic madness (38), locura manganica (describing a hypomanic syndrome of Chilean miners) (139), and manganese mania (140).

Although many of these victims have been misdiagnosed as schizophrenic, the most dramatic symptoms have been manic in nature with mental excitement, aggressive behavior, and incoherent speech as prominent features (141). Depression is less dramatic but has been reported in an even larger proportion of manganese-toxic persons (142). Other psychiatric symptoms include extreme irritability, insomnia, refusing food, and spontaneous laughing and crying at inappropriate moments.

The earliest signs of manganese poisoning are usually a generalized severe malaise and psychiatric signs. This is not surprising because manganese poisoning causes destruction of the nigro striatal areas of the basal ganglia in the brain. Diagnosis is established by quantitative serum levels greater than 0.05 ppm or elevated brain levels (38).

Bismuth. Psychiatric symptomatology has been reported in France and Australia as a consequence of oral bismuth, which is used in those countries for a variety of gastrointestinal disorders. Many cases are unrecognized in the United States because bismuth can be absorbed transdermally. It is a major component of many skin lightening creams and most doctors are unaware of that fact.

Two phases of toxicity are described. First, an insidious period lasting 1 to 8 weeks in which psychiatric symptoms including depression, anxiety, apathy, slowed mentation, and delusions are prominent (3, 38, 143, 144). Acute onset of a myoclonic encephalopathy is a sign of progression and may include four separate clinical pictures: 1) a severe organic brain syndrome similar to delirium tremens including fluctuating states of consciousness and terrifying visual hallucination; 2) abnormal movements including myoclonic jerks and an intention pseudo tremor; 3) problems standing and walking; and 4) language problems including disarthria, which sometimes degenerates to a babble (3, 143, 144). There is also a distinctive EEG pattern of 3 to 5 Hz, monomorphic waves, and a diffuse low voltage beta rhythm (144). Diagnosis is confirmed by demonstration of elevated blood and urine bismuth levels. Prognosis is excellent after stopping bismuth administration; improvement usually occurs within 3 to 10 weeks.

Thallium. Thallium poisoning was much more common in the past when it was used as a treatment for ringworm, syphilis, and as a depilatory agent. It continued to be used in rat and insect poisons in the United States until the 1970s when it was banned. It is still available in other countries and most poisonings today are the result of suicide or homicide attempts or accidental ingestion. Psychiatric symptoms can include psychosis and hallucinations; depressive symptoms can include decreased concentration, irritability, fatigue, and anorexia. All symptoms are usually accompanied by alopecia and gastrointestinal distress (38, 145, 146).

Aluminum. Dialysis dementia is a disorder recently linked to elevated aluminum levels (147–154). It occurs only among patients on hemodialysis. It is characterized by speech disorder with speech arrest, dysarthria, dysphasia, myoclonic epilepsy, abnormal EEG, partial complex and generalized seizures, and progressive mental deterioration terminating in advanced dementia (149). Behavioral or mental changes ranging from decreased memory to severe depression and even hallucination can occur as the first sign of dialysis dementia in 21 to 25 percent of patients. In one study (149), 86 percent of the patients eventually developed psychiatric symptoms that were misdiagnosed and incorrectly and unsuccessfully treated as major depression with tricyclic antidepressants. This occurred frequently until the true toxic nature of this disorder was uncovered (148, 149) and dialysis fluids were changed to lower aluminum content.

Tin (Organic Tins).   Dimethyltin dichloride, methyl chloride, and trimethyltin chloride are a class of compounds called organotins because they contain a complex of tin and an organic molecule. Psychiatric symptoms were reported after an industrial accident and include reported bouts of severe depression of short duration alternating with unprovoked attacks of temper and rate (155).

Magnesium.   Hypermagnesiumia may cause lassitude, depression, and a psychotic and a nonpsychotic organic brain syndrome that resolves as serum levels normalize (38).

Copper.   Wilson's disease, a disorder of copper metabolism that results in diffuse copper deposition throughout the body, is well known to cause symptoms indistinguishable from depression to bipolar disorder and schizophrenia. Simultaneous demonstrations of decreased serum copper and decreased ceruloplasmin is diagnostic even in the absence of a Kaiser-Fleisher Ring. Acquired copper toxicity is reported but no psychiatric symptoms have been noted; instead, the hematologic, gastrointestinal, and cardiovascular systems are affected (6, 156).

Vanadium.   Vanadium poisoning has been noted to cause depression and melancholia in Polish miners (157). Dick et al. (158) demonstrated significantly elevated vanadium plasma levels in depressed and bipolar manic patients as compared to normal controls. Depressed and bipolar manic patients treated with low vanadium diets showed significant improvement in their disorders (159).

Cadmium.   Elevated hair cadmium levels have been suggested as being etiologically related to the development of learning disabilities in children (160).

Bromism.   Bromide preparations were widely used as anticonvulsants and sedative hypnotics in the past. Although they are now outmoded and seldom seen today, psychiatric side effects were well known to occur 40 to 50 years ago. Milder psychiatric symptoms are more likely to appear at lower serum levels of 6 meq/L (50 mg percent) to 19 mq/L (150 mg percent) (3, 161). They include confusion, drowsiness, inability to concentrate, fatigue, malaise, and depression. Higher serum levels of 12 to 19 meq/L can cause more severe symptoms, including extreme agitation and excitement requiring sedation and restraint and psychosis including thought disorder, delusions, and auditory and visual hallucinations. Although the psychosis was labeled schizophrenic in the past, many cases appear to be indistinguishable from bipolar manic or schizoaffective disorder under today's diagnostic criteria (161–163). Patients can also develop a severe delirium characterized by fluctuating states of consciousness and mood (163). From a high of 21 percent bromide-related psychiatric hospital admissions in 1927 (164), the rates have steadily declined over the years to 5 to 16 percent in 1938 (161), 5 percent in 1940 (165), and 1 percent in 1965 (166), and are now reduced to sporadic case reports.

ANTICHOLINESTERASE, ORGANOPHOSPHATE INSECTICIDES, AND NERVE GASES

Organophosphate insecticides, nerve gases used in chemical warfare, and drugs used to treat myasthenia gravis act by inhibiting the enzyme acetylcholinesterase in either a reversible or permanent manner. Normal individuals exposed to these agents rapidly develop irritability, tension, anxiety, jitteriness, restlessness, giddiness, emotional withdrawal, depression, drowsiness, decreased concentration, confusion, and unusual dreams (167–169).

Increased anxiety (170, 171), depression (172), and decreased memory and attention (172, 173) can result when individuals are chronically exposed to organophosphate insecticides. Early reports of schizophrenic symptoms have not been substantiated (172).

CARBON MONOXIDE

Carbon monoxide is a nonirritating colorless, odorless gas. It has 200 times more affinity for the oxygen-carrying hemoglobin site than oxygen itself. Carbon monoxide poisoning produces hypoxia through the body, thus selectively affecting brain functioning.

The psychiatric and neurologic consequences of carbon monoxide poisoning occur in a bimodal pattern immediately after exposure or may be delayed as much as 1 to 3 weeks. The symptoms can fluctuate so much that carbon monoxide poisoning has been misdiagnosed as hysterical psychosis, borderline personality, schizophrenia, psychotic depression, catatonia, and hysteria. Electroconvulsive therapy is contraindicated. Carboxyhemoglobin should be measured in all suspected cases.

CARBON DIOXIDE

Carbon dioxide has recently been used to induce panic attacks in panic-disordered individuals.

VOLATILE SUBSTANCES

Today two groups are exposed to volatile hydrocarbons and subsequently develop psychiatric symptoms. The best studied group consists of persons who are exposed to these substances occupationally, such as painters, refinery workers, and persons who fuel airplanes. Acute effects depend on dose and include euphoria, excitation, auditory and visual hallucinations, and bizarre behavior at low doses. Higher doses can progress from confusion and disorientation to stupor and coma (174). Long-term effects are dependent on many years' duration of exposure and include decreased short memory and increased reaction times (175), personality changes, irritability, anxiety, panic disorder symptoms, somatic complaints, fatigue, depression, and organic brain syndromes (176–178).

The other group, less well studied, consists of children and adolescents who intentionally abuse glue, toluene, gasoline, cleaning fluid (trichloroethane), and nitrous oxide in order to experience those substances' euphorigenic effects. Immediate effects include euphoria, hallucination (in 50 percent of cases), and conduct disordered behavior (174).

APPROACH TO THE INDIVIDUAL

The previous discussion makes it clear that there are no pathognomic signs or symptoms of a medication-induced or toxin-induced disorder. It is very important, therefore, to be aware of this class of disorder and to maintain a high index of suspicion, to ask appropriate historical and occupational questions, to perform appropriate laboratory tests, and to observe the patient in as drug-free a state as possible. When confronted with a patient manifesting psychiatric or behavioral symptoms, the best approach to diagnosing medication- or toxin-induced psychiatric disorders is to perform that evaluation as part of an integrated structured approach to the patient.

Every psychiatric patient should go through a drug-free wash-out period for 1 to 2 weeks if possible. If some medications are necessary to preserve life or psychiatric or behavioral control, the least toxic substitutes available should be used.

A comprehensive, supervised urine (i.e., direct urethral visualization) drug-of-abuse screen using antibody-based immunoassay, gas chromatography, or GC/MS (but not thin layer chromotography) is mandatory. All prescribed medications should be monitored by measuring the appropriate blood levels. This can help reveal both the degree of patient medication compliance as well as detect toxic levels that developed accidentally or resulted from an intentional suicide overdose. Whatever the cause, elevated medication or toxin levels can produce psychiatric side effects.

A careful detailed occupational history is frequently ignored, but it is critical because it can reveal exposure to many of the industrial or environmental toxins mentioned earlier in this chapter. If the individual was indeed exposed, appropriate blood and urine testing can be ordered.

If none of these examinations prove to be successful, a medical illness presenting with psychiatric symptoms is another possibility that also needs to be ruled out before any definitive psychiatric treatment is started. Throughout these examinations the evaluating psychiatrist must continually ask questions such as "Why is this individual particularly vulnerable to the development of psychiatric symptoms?" and "What have I missed, forgotten, or overlooked?"

If any particular medication or toxin is identified as the cause of the psychiatric symptoms, exposure must be stopped or the offending agent must be removed from the environment. Often gradual improvement and clearing of the psychiatric side effects occurs when this is accomplished. Sometimes, after an appropriate period of time has elapsed and no improvement has taken place, judicious institution of psychiatric treatments aimed at eliminating the residual psychiatric symptomatology may be necessary.

REFERENCES

1. Hall RCW, Gardner ER, Popkin MK, Lecann AF, Stickney SK: Unrecognized physical illness prompting psychiatric admission: a prospective study. Am J Psychiatry 138:629–635, 1981

2. Hall RCW, Popkin MK, Devaul RA, Faillance LA, Stickney SK: Physical illness presenting as psychiatric disease. Arch Gen Psychiatry 35:1315–1320, 1978

3. Jefferson JW, Marshall JR: Neuropsychiatric Features of Medical Disorders. New York, Plenum Press, 1981

4. Koranyi EK: Morbidity and rate of undiagnosed physical illness in a psychiatric clinic population. Arch Gen Psychiatry 36:414–419, 1979

5. Klein DF, Gittelman R, Quitkin F, Rifkin A: Diagnosis and Drug Treatment of Psychiatric Disorders: Adults and Children. Baltimore, Williams & Wilkins, 1980

6. Estroff TW, Gold MS: Psychiatric misdiagnosis, in Advances in Psychopharmacology: Predicting and Improving Treatment Response. Edited by Gold MS, Lydiard RB, Carman JS. Boca Raton, Florida, CRC Press Inc, 1984

7. American Psychiatric Association: Diagnostic and Statistical Manual of Mental Disorders. 3rd ed. American Psychiatric Association, Washington, DC, 1980

8. Anonymous: Drugs that cause psychiatric symptoms. The Medical Letter 23:9–12, 1981

9. Hall RCW, Stickney SK, Gardner ER: Behavioral toxicity of nonpsychiatric drugs, in Psychiatric Presentations of Medical Illness: Somatopsychic Disorders. Edited by Hall RCW. New York, Spectrum Publications, 1980

9a. Spitzer RL, Endicott J, Robins E: Research Diagnostic Criteria (RDC) for a Selected Group of Functional Disorders. New York, New York State Psychiatric Institute, 1980

10. Boston Collaborative Drug-Related Programs: Psychiatric side effects of non-psychiatric drugs. Sem Psychiat 3:406–420, 1971

11. Goodwin FK: Behavioral effects of L-dopa in man. Seminars in Psychiatry 3:477–492, 1971

12. Goodwin FK, Bunney WE: Depressions following reserpine: a reevaluation. Seminars in Psychiatry 3:435–448, 1971

13. Paykel ES, Fleminger R, Watson JP: Psychiatric side effects of antihypertensive drugs other than reserpine. J Clin Pharmacol 2:14–39, 1982

14. Fingl E, Woodbury DM: General principles, in The Pharmacologic Basis of Therapeutics. 8th ed. Edited by Goodman LS, Gillman A. New York, Macmillan, 1980

15. Angrist B, Sudilovsky A: Central nervous system stimulants: historical aspects and clinical effects, in Handbook of Psychopharmacology. Edited by Iverson LI, Iverson SD, Snyder SH. New York, Plenum Press, 1978

16. Griffith JD, Cavanaugh JH, Held J, et al: Experimental psychosis induced by the administration of a d-amphetamine, in Amphetamines and Related Compounds. Edited by Costa E, Garattini S. New York, Raven Press, 1970, pp. 897–904

17. Griffith JD, Cavanaugh J, Held J, et al: Dextroamphetamine: evaluation of psychotomimetic properties in man. Arch Gen Psychiatry 26:97–100, 1972

18. Preskorn SH, Denner LJ: Benzodiazepines and withdrawal psychosis. JAMA 237:36–38, 1977

19. Dysken MW, Chan CH: Diazepam withdrawal psychosis: a case report. Am J Psychiatry 134:573, 1977

20. DeBard ML: Diazepam withdrawal syndrome: a case with psychosis, seizure and coma. Am J Psychiatry 136:104–105, 1979

21. Flemenbaum A, Gunby B: Ethchlorvynol (Placidyl) abuse and withdrawal (review of clinical picture and report of 2 cases). Diseases of the Nervous System 32:188–192, 1971

22. Heston LL, Hastings D: Psychosis with withdrawal from ethchlorvynol. Am J Psychiatry 137:249–250, 1980

23. Holinger PC, Klawans HL: Reversal of tricyclic-overdosage-induced central anticholinergic syndrome by physostigmine. Am J Psychiatry 133:1018–1023, 1976

24. Siris SG, Van Kammen DP, Docherty JP: The use of antidepressant drugs in schizophrenia. Arch Gen Psychiatry 35:1368–1377, 1978

25. Sheehy LM, Maxmen JS: Phenelzine-induced psychosis. Am J Psychiatry 135:1422–1423, 1978

26. Kramer JC, Klein DF, Fink M: Withdrawal symptoms following discontinuation of imipramine therapy. Am J Psychiatry 118:549–550, 1961

27. Moreines R, Gold MS: MAO inhibitors: predicting response/maximizing efficacy, in Advances in Psychopharmacology: Predicting and Improving Treatment Response. Edited by Gold MS, Lydiard RB, Carman JS. Boca Raton, Florida, CRC Press Inc, 1984

28. Behrman S: Mutism induced by phenothiazines. Br J Psychiatry 121:559–604, 1972

29. Williams P: An unusual response to chlorpromazine therapy. Br J Psychiatry 121:439–440, 1972

30. Gelenberg AJ: The catatonic syndrome. Lancet 1:1339–1341, 1976

31. Gardos G, Cole JO, Tarsy D: Withdrawal syndromes associated with antipsychotic drugs. Am J Psychiatry 135:1321–1324, 1978

32. Van Putten T, May PRA: Akinetic depression in schizophrenia. Arch Gen Psychiatry 35:1101–1107, 1978

33. Mueller PS, Vester JW, Fermaglich J: Neuroleptic malignant syndrome: successful treatment with bromocriptine. JAMA 249:386–388, 1983

34. Scarlett JD, Zimmerman R, Berkovic SF: Neuroleptic malignant syndrome. Aust NZ J Med 13:70–73, 1983

35. Perl M, Hall RCW, Gardner ER: Behavioral toxicity of psychiatric drugs, in Psychiatric Presentations of Medical Illness. Edited by Hall RCW. New York, Spectrum Publications, 1980

36. Bajor GF: Memory loss with lithium? Am J Psychiatry 134:588, 1977

37. Rifkin A, Quitkin F, Klein DF: Organic brain syndrome during lithium carbonate treatment. Compr Psychiatry 14:251–254, 1973

38. Edwards N: Mental disturbances related to metals, in Psychiatric Presentations of Medical Illness. Edited by Hall RCW. New York, Spectrum Publications, 1980

39. Sellers J. Tyre RP, Whiteley A, et al: Neurotoxic effects of lithium with delayed rise in serum lithium levels. Br J Psychiatry 140:623–625, 1982

40. Donaldson IMG, Cuningham J: Persisting neurologic sequelae of lithium carbonate therapy. Arch Neurol 40:747–751, 1983

41. Rainey JM: Disulfiram toxicity and carbon disulfide poisoning. Am J Psychiatry 134:371–378, 1977

42. Liddon SC, Satran R: Disulfiram (Antabuse) psychosis. Am J Psychiatry 123:1284–1289, 1967

43. Knee ST, Razani J: Acute organic brain syndrome: a complication of disulfiram therapy. Am J Psychiatry 131:1281–1282, 1974

44. Quail M, Karelse RH: Disulfiram psychosis: a case report. Afr Med J 57:551–552, 1980

45. Goodwin FK, Ebert MH, Bunney WE: Mental effects of reserpine in man: a review, in Psychiatric Complications of Medical Drugs. Edited by Shader RI. New York, Raven Press, 1972

46. Muller JC, Pryor WW, Gibbons JE: Depression and anxiety occurring during rauwolfia therapy. JAMA 159:836–839, 1955

47. Fries ED: Mental depression in hypertensive patients treated for long periods with large doses of reserpine. N Engl J Med 251:1006–1008, 1954

48. Jensen K: Depressions in patients treated with reserpine for arterial hypertension. Acta Psychiatr Neurol Scand 34:195–204, 1959

49. Schroeder HA, Perry HM: Psychosis apparently produced by reserpine. JAMA 159:839–840, 1955

50. Hawkins DJ: Acute organic brain syndrome psychosis with methyldopa therapy. Mo Med 73: 476–481, 1976

51. Turner WM: Lidocaine and psychotic reactions. Ann Intern Med 97:149–150, 1982

52. McCrum ID, Guidry JR: Procainamide-induced psychosis. JAMA 240:1265–1266, 1978

53. Padfield PL, Smith DA, Fitzsimos EJ, et al: Disopyramide and acute psychosis. Lancet 1:1152, 1977

54. Falk RH, Nisbet PA, Gray TJ: Mental distress in patients on disopyramide. Lancet 1:858–859, 1977

55. Ahmad S, Sheikh AI, Meeran MK: Disopyramide-induced acute psychosis. Chest 76:712, 1979

56. Duroziez P: De delire et du coma digitaliques. Gazette Hebdonadaire de Medecine et de Chirurgie 11:780–783, 1874

57. Marriott HJL: Delirium from digitalis toxicity. JAMA 203:178, 1968

58. Church G, Marriott JHL: Digitalis delirium: a report on three cases. Circulation 20:549–553, 1959

59. Volpe BT, Soave R: Formed visual hallucinations as digitalis toxicity. Ann Intern Med 91:865–866, 1979

60. Gorelick DA, Kussin SZ, Kahn I: Single case study paranoid delusions and auditory hallucinations associated with digoxin intoxication. J Nerv Ment Dis 166:817–818, 1978

61. Shear MK, Sacks MH: Digitalis delirium: report of two cases. Am J Psychiatry 135:109–110, 1978

62. Tollefson G: Psychiatric implications of anticonvulsant drugs. J Clin Psychiatry 41:295–302, 1980

63. Stores G: Behavioural effects of anti-epileptic drugs. Develop Med Child Neurol 17:647–658, 1975

64. Franks RD, Richter AJ: Schizophrenia-like psychosis associated with anticonvulsant toxicity. Am J Psychiatry 136:873–974, 1979

65. Glaser GH: Diphenylhydantoin toxicity, in Antiepileptic Drugs. Edited by Woodbury DM, Penry JK, Schmidt RP. New York, Raven Press, 1972

66. Booker HE: Primidone toxicity, in Antiepileptic Drugs. Edited by Woodbury DM, Penry JK, Schmidt RP. New York, Raven Press, 1972

67. Roger J, Grangeon H, Guey J, Lob H: Psychological and psychiatric symptoms in treatment of epileptics with ethosuccimide. Encephale 57:407–438, 1968

68. Buchanan RA: Ethosuximide toxicity, in Antiepileptic Drugs. Edited by Woodbury DM, Penry JK, Schmidt RP. New York, Raven Press, 1972

69. Dalby MA: Antiepileptic and psychotropic effects of carbamazepine (Tegretol) in the treatment of psychomotor epilepsy. Epilepsia 12:325–334, 1971

70. Jones RF, Lance JW: Baclofen (Lioresal) in the long-term management of spasticity. Med J Aust 1:654–657, 1976

71. Skausig OB, Korsgaard S: Hallucinations and baclofen. Lancet 1:1258, 1977

72. Arnold ES, Rudd SM, Kirshner H: Manic psychosis following rapid withdrawal from baclofen. Am J Psychiatry 137:1466–1467, 1980

73. Lees AJ, Clarke CRA, Harrison MJ: Hallucinations after withdrawal of baclofen. Lancet 1:858, 1977

74. Presthus J, Holmsen R: Appraisal of long-term levodopa treatment of parkinsonism with special reference to therapy limiting factors. Acta Neurol Scand 50:774–790, 1974

75. Moskovitz C, Moses H, Klawans HL: Levodopa-induced psychosis: a kindling phenomenon. Am J Psychiatry 135:669–675, 1978

76. Parkes D: Mechanisms of bromocriptine-induced hallucinations. N Engl J Med 302:1479, 1979

77. Goodkin DA: Mechanisms of bromocriptine-induced hallucinations. N Engl J Med 302:1479, 1979

78. Calne DB, Plotkin C, Williams AC, et al: Long-term treatment of parkinsonism with bromocriptine. Lancet 1:735–738, 1978

79. Vlissides DN, Gill D, Castelow J: Bromocriptine-induced mania? Br Med J [Clin Res] 1:510, 1978

80. Weiner N: Atropine, scopolamine and related anti-muscarinic drugs, in The Pharmacological Basis of Therapeutics. Edited by Gillman AG, Goodman LS, Gillman A. New York, Macmillan, 1980, pp 120–137

81. Hall RCW, Popkin MK, McHenry LE: Angel's trumpet psychosis: a central nervous system anticholinergic syndrome. Am J Psychiatry 134:312–314, 1977

82. Brizer DA, Manning DW: Delirium induced by poisoning with anticholinergic agents. Am J Psychiatry 139:1343–1344, 1982

83. Gotz V: Paranoid psychosis with indomethacin. Br Med J 1:49, 1978

84. Katz AM, Pearson CM, Kennedy JM: A clinical trial of indomethacin in rheumatoid arthritis. Clin Pharmacol Ther 6:25–30, 1965

85. Carney MWP: Paranoid psychosis with indomethacin. Br Med J 2:994–995, 1977

86. Thompson M, Percy JS: Further experience with indomethacin in the treatment of rheumatic disorders. Br Med J 1:80–83, 1966

87. Rothermich NO: An extended study of indomethacin: I. Clinical pharmacology. JAMA 195:123–128, 1966

88. Kruis R, Barger R: Paranoid psychosis with sulindac. JAMA 243:1420, 1980

89. Thornton TL: Delirium associated with sulindac. JAMA 243:1630–1631, 1980

90. Peterson LG, Popkin MK: Neuropsychiatric effects of chemotherapeutic agents for cancer. Psychosomatics 21:141–153, 1980

91. Stolinsky DC, Bogdon DL, Solomon J, et al: Hexamethylamine (NSC 13875) alone and in combination with 5-(3, 3-dimethyl-1-triazeno) imidazole-4-carboxamide (NSC-45388). Treatment of Advanced Cancer 30:654–659, 1972

92. Kay HEM, Knapton PJ, O'Sullivan JP, et al: Encephalopathy in acute leukemia associated with methotrexate therapy. Arch Dis Child 47:344–354, 1972

93. Holland J, Fasanello S, Ohnuma T: Psychiatric symptoms associated with L-asparaginase administration. J Psychiatr Res 10:105–113, 1974

94. Moure JMB, Whitecar JP, Bodey GP: Electroencephalogram changes secondary to asparaginase. Arch Neurol 23:265–368, 1970

95. Carbone PP, Haskell CM, Leventhal BG, et al: Clinical experience with L-asparaginase. Recent Results Cancer Res 33:236–243, 1970

96. Mann AM, Hutchinson JR: Manic reaction associated with procarbazine hydrochloride therapy of Hodgkin's disease. Can Med Assoc J 97:1350–1353, 1967

97. Hamilton RC, Dundee JW, Clarke RSJ, et al: Studies of drugs given before anesthesia XIII: Pentazocine and other opiate antagonists. Br J Anaesth 39:647–656, 1967

98. Eckenhoff JE, Kneale DH, Dripps RD: The incidence and etiology of postanesthetic excitement. Anesthesiology 22:667–673, 1961

99. Davison LA, Steinhelber JC, Eger EI, et al: Psychological effects of halothane and isoflurane anesthesia. Anesthesiology 43:313–324, 1975

100. Selikoff IJ, Robitzek EH, Ornstein CG: Toxicity of hydrazine derivatives of isonicotinic acid in the chemotherapy of human tuberculosis. Quarterly Bulletin of Sea View Hospital 13:17–26, 1952

101. Chu J: Toxic psychosis due to overdosage of isonicotinic acid hydrazide. Va Med J 49:125–127, 1953

102. Hunter RA: Confusional psychosis with residual organic cerebral impairment following isoniazid therapy. Lancet 2:960–962, 1952

103. Kiersch TA: Toxic organic psychoses due to isoniazid therapy. US Armed Forces Medical Journal 5:1353–1359, 1954

104. Wallach MB, Gershon S: Psychiatric sequelae to tuberculosis chemotherapy, in Psychiatric Complications of Medical Drugs. Edited by Shader RI. New York, Raven Press, 1972

105. McConnell RB, Cheetham HD: Acute pellagra during isoniazid therapy. Lancet 2:959–960, 1952

106. Lewis WC, Calden G, Thurston JR, et al: Psychiatric and neurological reactions to cycloserine in the treatment of tuberculosis. Diseases of the Chest 32:172–182, 1957

107. Bjornberg A, Selstam J: Acute psychotic reaction after injection of procaine penicillin: a report of 33 cases. Acta Psychiatr Neurol Scand 35:129–139, 1959

108. Eggleston DJ: Procaine penicillin psychosis. Br Dent J 148:73–74, 1980

109. Green RL, Lewis JE, Kraus SJ, et al: Elevated plasma procaine concentrations after administration of procaine penicillin G. N Engl J Med 291:223–226, 1974

110. Winn RE, Bower MJ, Richards MJ: Acute toxic delirium neurotoxicity of intrathecal administration of amphotericin B. Arch Intern Med 139:706–707, 1979

111. Torrey EF: Chloroquine seizures: report of four cases. JAMA 204:115–118, 867–870, 1968

112. Engel GL: Quinacrine effects on the central nervous system. JAMA 197:235, 1966

113. Flind AC, Jones DR: Mental confusion and cimetidine. Lancet 1:379, 1979

114. Grimson TA: Reactions to cimetidine. Lancet 1:858, 1977

115. Beraud JJ, Monteil AL, Munoz A, et al: Confusion mentale au cours d'un traitement par la cimetidine. Nouvelle Presse Medical 7:29, 1978

116. Agarwal SK: Cimetidine and visual hallucinations. JAMA 240:214, 1978

117. Kimelblatt BJ, Cerra FB, Calleri G, et al: Dose and serum concentration relationships in cimetidine associated mental confusion. Gastroenterology 78:791–795, 1980

118. Nouel O, Bernuau J, Lebar M, et al: Cimetidine-induced mental confusion in patients with cirrhosis. Gastroenterology 79:780–781, 1980

119. Adler LE, Sadja L, Wilets G: Cimetidine toxicity manifested as paranoia and hallucinations. Am J Psychiatry 137:1112–1113, 1980

120. Barnhart CC, Bowden CL: Toxic psychosis with cimetidine. Am J Psychiatry 136:725–726, 1979

121. Arneson GA: More on toxic psychosis with cimetidine. Am J Psychiatry 136:1348–1349, 1979

122. Jefferson JW: Central nervous system toxicity of cimetidine: a case of depression. Am J Psychiatry 136:346, 1979

123. Needleman HL: The neuropsychiatric implications of low level exposure to lead. Psychol Med 12:461–463, 1982

124. Cullen MR, Robins JM, Eskenazi B: Adult inorganic lead intoxication presentation of 31 new cases and a review of recent advances in the literature. Medicine (Baltimore) 62:221–247, 1983

125. Baker EL, Feldman RG, White RF, et al: The role of occupational lead exposure in the genesis of psychiatric and behavioral disturbances. Acta Psychiatr Scand 67:38–48, 1983

126. Yule, W, Lansdown R, Millar IB, et al: The relationship between blood lead concentrations, intelligence and attainment in a school population: a pilot study. Dev Med Child Neurol 23:567–576, 1981

127. David OJ, Wintrob HL, Arcoleo CG: Blood lead stability. Arch Environ Health 37:147–150, 1982

128. David OJ, Hoffman SP, Sverd J, et al: Lead and hyperactivity: lead levels among hyperactive children. J Abnorm Child Psychol 5:405–416, 1977

129. Gittelman R, Eskenazi B: Lead and hyperactivity revisited: an investigation of nondisadvantaged children. Arch Gen Psychiatry 40:827–833, 1983

130. David OJ, Clark J, Voeller K: Lead and hyperactivity. Lancet 2:900–903, 1972

131. Landrigan PJ, Whitworth RH, Baloh RW, et al: Neuropsychological dysfunction in children with chronic low-level lead absorption. Lancet 1:708–712, 1975

132. Freeman JA: Mercurial disease among hatters. Transaction of the New Jersey State Medical Society 61:61–64, 1860

133. Maghazaji HI: Psychiatric aspects of methyl mercury poisoning. J Neurol Neurosurg Psychiatry 37:954–958, 1974

134. Cole M, Scheulein M, Kerwin DM: Arsenical encephalopathy due to the use of milibis. Arch Intern Med 117:706–711, 1966

135. Frank G: Neurologische und psychiarische folgesymptomie bei akuter arsen-wasserstoff-vergiftung. J Neurol 70:213–259, 1976

136. Jenkins RB: Inorganic arsenic and the nervous system. Brain 89:479–498, 1966

137. Harvey SC: Heavy metals, in The Pharmacological Basis of Therapeutics. Edited by Goodman LS, Gilman W. New York, Macmillan, 1975, pp 924–928

138. Freeman JW, Couch JR: Prolonged encephalopathy with arsenic poisoning. Neurology 28:853–855, 1978

139. Mena I, Marin O, Fuenzalida S, et al: Chronic manganese poisoning clinical picture and manganese turnover. Neurology 17:128–136, 1967

140. Rodier J, Manganese poisoning in Moroccan miners. Br J Ind Med 12:21–35, 1955

141. Chandra SV: Psychiatric illness due to manganese poisoning. Acta Psychiatr Scand 67:49–54, 1983

142. Abdel Naby S, Hassanein M: Neuropsychiatric manifestations of chronic manganese poisoning. J Neurol Neurosurg Psychiatry 28:282–288, 1965

143. Loiseau D, Henry P, Jallon P, et al: Atrogenic myollonic encephalopathies caused by bismuth salts. J Neurol Sci 27:133–143, 1976

144. Supino-Viterbo V, Sicard C, Riszegliato M, et al: Toxic encephalopathy due to ingestion of bismuth salts: clinical and EEG studies of 45 patients. J Neurol Neurosurg Psychiatry 40:748–752, 1977

145. Munch JC: Human thallotoxicosis. JAMA 102:1929–1934, 1984

146. Gruneeld O, Hinostroza G: Thallium poisoning. Arch Intern Med 114:132–138, 1964

147. Elliott HL: Dialysis dementia, in Metabolic Disorders of the Nervous System. Edited by Rose FC. London, Pitman, 1981, pp. 359–366

148. Dunea G, Mahurkar SD, Mamdani B, et al: Role of aluminum in dialysis dementia. Ann Intern Med 88:502–504, 1978

149. O'Hare JA, Callaghan NM, Murnaghan DJ: Dialysis encephalopathy: clinical, electroencephalographic and interventional aspects. Medicine 62:129–141, 1983

150. Arieff AI, Cooper JD, Armstrong D, et al: Dementia, renal failure, and brain aluminum. Ann Intern Med 90:741–747, 1979

151. Alfrey AC, Le Gendre GR, Kaehny DW: The dialysis encephalopathy syndrome: possible aluminum intoxication. N Engl J Med 294:184–188, 1976

152. Alfrey AC, Smythe WR: Trace element abnormalities in chronic uremia. Proceedings of the 11th Annual Contract Conference for Artificial Kidney and Chronic Uremia Progress, NIAMDD 11:103–104, 1978

153. McDermott JR, Smith AI, Ward MK, Parkinson JS, Kerr DNS: Brain-aluminum concentration in dialysis encephalopathy. Lancet 1:901–903, 1978

154. Elliott HL, Dryburgh F, Fell GS, Sabet S, MacDougall AI: Aluminium toxicity during regular haemodialysis. Br Med J 1:1101–1103, 1978

155. Ross WD, Emmett EA, Steiner J, et al: Neurotoxic effects of occupational exposure to organotins. Am J Psychiatry 138:1092–1095, 1981

156. Scheinberg IH: Neurological and behavioral aspects of Wilson's disease, in Electrolytes and Neuropsychiatric Disorders. Edited by Alexander PE. Lancaster, MTP Press, 1981, pp 113–120

157. Witkowska D, Brezinski J: Alteration of brain noradrenaline dopamine and 5 hydroxytryptamine levels during vanadium poisoning. Pol J Pharmacol Pharm 31:393–398, 1974

158. Dick DAT, Dick EG, Naylor GJ: Plasma Vanadium concentration in manic depressive illness. J Physiol (London) 310:27–31, 1981

159. Naylor GJ, Smith AHW: Vanadium: a possible *deteriological* factor in manic depressive illness. Psychol Med 11:249–256, 1981

160. Pihl RO, Markes M: Hair element content in learning disabled children. Science 198:204–206, 1977

161. Hanes FM, Yates A: An analysis of four hundred instances of chronic bromide intoxication. South Med J 31:667–671, 1938

162. Levin M: Bromide psychosis: four varieties. Am J Psychiatry 104:798–800, 1948

163. Perkins HA: Bromide intoxication. Arch Intern Med 85:783–794, 1950

164. Wuth O: Rational bromide treatment. JAMA 88:2013–2017, 1927

165. Anonymous: Hazards of bromidism in proprietary and uncontrolled hypnotic medication: Neurosine (Dios Chemical Company) not acceptable for N.N.R.: report of the council on pharmacy and chemistry. JAMA 115:933, 1940

166. Ewing JA, Grand WJ: The bromide hazard. South Med J 58:148–152, 1965

167. Grob D, Harvey A: The effects and treatment of nerve gas poisoning. Am J Med 14:52–63, 1953

168. Rountree DW, Nevin S, Wilson A: The effects of diisopropylfluorophosphonate in schizophrenia and manic-depressive psychosis. J Neurol Neurosurg Psychiatry 13:472–478, 1950

169. Bowers MB, Goodman E, Sim VM: Some behavioral changes in man following anticholinesterase administration. J Nerv Ment Dis 138:383–389, 1964

170. Levin HS, Rodnitzky RL, Mick DL: Anxiety associated with exposure to organophosphate compounds. Arch Gen Psychiatry 33:225–228, 1976

171. Dille JR, Smith TW: Central nervous system effects of chronic exposure to organophosphate insecticides. Aerospace Medicine 35:475–478, 1964

172. Gershon S, Shaw FH: Psychiatric sequelae of chronic exposure to organophosphorus insecticides. Lancet 1:1371–1374, 1961

173. Durham WF, Wolfe HR, Quinby GE: Organophosphorus insecticides and mental alertness. Arch Environ Health 10:55–66, 1965

174. Wyse DG: Deliberate inhalation of volatile hypocarbons: a review. Can Med Assoc J 108:71–74, 1973

175. Lindstrom K, Wickstrom G: Psychological function changes among maintenance house painters exposed to low levels of organic solvent mixtures. Acta Psychiatr Scand 67:81–91, 1983

176. Struwe G, Knave B, Mindus P: Neuropsychiatric symptoms in workers exposed to jet fuel—a combined epidemiological and causistic study. Acta Psychiatr Scand 67:55–67, 1983

177. Capurro PU, Capurro C: Solvent exposure and mental depression. Clinical Toxicology 15:193–195, 1979

178. Struwe G, Wennberg A: Psychiatric and neurological symptoms in workers occupationally exposed to organic solvents—results of a differential epidemiological study. Acta Psychiatr Scand 67:68–80, 1983